# Cosmetic Rhinoplasty

*Guest Editor*

MINAS CONSTANTINIDES, MD, FACS

# FACIAL PLASTIC SURGERY CLINICS OF NORTH AMERICA

www.facialplastic.theclinics.com

February 2009 • Volume 17 • Number 1

SAUNDERS an imprint of ELSEVIER, Inc.

**W.B. SAUNDERS COMPANY**
*A Division of Elsevier Inc.*

1600 John F. Kennedy Blvd., Suite 1800, Philadelphia, PA 19103-2899

http://www.theclinics.com

**FACIAL PLASTIC SURGERY CLINICS OF NORTH AMERICA Volume 17, Number 1**
**February 2009 ISSN 1064-7406, ISBN 1-4377-0473-5, 978-1-4377-0473-0**

Editor: Joanne Husovski
Developmental Editor: Donald Mumford

*Facial Plastic Surgery Clinics of North America* (ISSN 1064-7406) is published quarterly by Elsevier Inc., 360 Park Avenue South, New York, NY 10010-1710. Months of issue are February, May, August, and November. Business and Editorial Offices: 1600 John F. Kennedy Blvd., Suite 1800, Philadelphia, PA 19103-2899. Periodicals postage paid at New York, NY, and additional mailing offices. Subscription prices are $273.00 per year (US individuals), $428.00 per year (US institutions), $307.00 per year (Canadian individuals), $513.00 per year (Canadian institutions), $368.00 per year (foreign individuals), $513.00 per year (foreign institutions), $133.00 per year (US students), and $185.00 per year (foreign students). Foreign air speed delivery is included in all *Clinics* subscription prices. All prices are subject to change without notice. POSTMASTER: Send address changes to *Facial Plastic Surgery Clinics*, Elsevier Periodicals Customer Service, 11830 Westline Industrial Drive, St. Louis, MO 63146. **Customer service: 1-800-654-2452 (US and Canada); 1-314-453-7041 (outside US and Canada); Fax: 314-453-5170; E-mail: journalscustomerservice-usa@elsevier.com (for print support); journalsonlinesupport-usa@elsevier.com (for online support).**

*Reprints*. For copies of 100 or more of articles in this publication, please contact the Commercial Reprints Department, Elsevier Inc., 360 Park Avenue South, New York, NY 10010-1710. Tel.: 212-633-3812; Fax: 212-462-1935; E-mail: reprints@elsevier.com.

*Facial Plastic Surgery Clinics of North America* is covered in *MEDLINE/PubMed* (*Index Medicus*).

Printed and bound by CPI Group (UK) Ltd, Croydon, CR0 4YY

Transferred to Digital Print 2011

# Contributors

## CONSULTING EDITOR

**J. REGAN THOMAS, MD**
Lederer Professor and Chairman, Department
of Otolaryngology—Head and Neck Surgery,
University of Illinois at Chicago College of
Medicine, Chicago, Illinois

## EDITORIAL BOARD

**SHAN R. BAKER, MD**
Professor and Chief, Section of Plastic
and Reconstructive Surgery, University
of Michigan, Ann Arbor, Michigan

**ROBERT KELLMAN, MD**
Professor and Chairman, Department
of Otolaryngology, State University of New
York Upstate Medical University, Syracuse,
New York

**RUSSELL W.H. KRIDEL, MD**
Clinical Associate Professor, Department of
Otolaryngology—Head and Neck Surgery,
Division of Facial Plastic Surgery, University of
Texas Health Science Center, Houston, Texas

**STEPHEN W. PERKINS, MD**
Private Practitioner, Perkins Facial Plastic
Surgery, Indianapolis, Indiana

**ANTHONY P. SCLAFANI, MD, FACS**
Director of Facial Plastic Surgery, The New
York Eye and Ear Infirmary, New York,
New York; and Professor of Otolaryngology—
Head and Neck Surgery, New York Medical
College, Valhalla, New York

## GUEST EDITOR

**MINAS CONSTANTINIDES, MD, FACS**
Director, Division of Facial Plastic and
Reconstructive Surgery, Department of
Otolaryngology–Head and Neck Surgery, New
York University School of Medicine, New York,
New York

## AUTHORS

**PETER A. ADAMSON, MD, FRCSC, FACS**
Professor and Head, Division of Facial Plastic
and Reconstructive Surgery, Department of
Otolaryngology–Head and Neck Surgery,
University of Toronto, Toronto, Ontario, Canada

**SHAN R. BAKER, MD**
Professor, Department of Otolaryngology,
Director, Center for Facial Cosmetic Surgery,
University of Michigan, Livonia, Michigan

**MICHAEL J. BRENNER, MD**
Assistant Professor of Surgery, Division
of Otolaryngology–Head & Neck Surgery,
Department of Surgery, Southern Illinois
University School of Medicine, Springfield, Illinois

**MARK A. CHECCONE, MD**
Assistant Professor, Department of
Otolaryngology–Head and Neck Surgery,
Washington University in St. Louis School
of Medicine, St. Louis, Missouri

**J. JARED CHRISTOPHEL, MD**
Chief Resident, Department of
Otolaryngology–Head and Neck Surgery,
University of Virginia Health System,
Charlottesville, Virginia

**MINAS CONSTANTINIDES, MD, FACS**
Director, Division of Facial Plastic and
Reconstructive Surgery; Department of
Otolaryngology–Head and Neck Surgery,
New York University School of Medicine,
New York, New York

**ETAI FUNK, MD**
The Bressler Center for Facial Plastic Surgery
and Skin Care; and Associate Clinical
Professor, Bobby R. Alford Department of
Otolaryngology–Head and Neck Surgery,
Baylor College of Medicine, Houston, Texas

**PETER A. HILGER, MD, FACS**
Director, Professor, Division of Facial Plastic
and Reconstructive Surgery; and Professor,
Department of Otolaryngology–Head & Neck
Surgery, University of Minnesota School of
Medicine, Minneapolis, Minnesota

**YONG JU. JANG, MD**
Professor, Department of Otolaryngology,
Asan Medical Center, University of Ulsan
College of Medicine, Songpa-gu, Seoul, Korea

**DAVID W. KIM, MD**
Chief, Division of Facial Plastic and
Reconstructive Surgery; and Associate
Professor, Department of Otolaryngology,
Head and Neck Surgery, University of
California, University of California, San
Francisco, California

**SAM P. MOST, MD**
Division of Facial Plastic and Reconstructive
Surgery, Stanford University School
of Medicine, Stanford, California

**STEPHEN S. PARK, MD, FACS**
Director, Division of Facial Plastic and
Reconstructive Surgery; and Vice Chairman,
Department of Otolaryngology–Head and Neck
Surgery, University of Virginia Health System,
Charlottesville, Virginia

**AMIT PATEL, MD**
Fellow, Meridian Plastic Surgeons and Medical
Skin Care, Indianapolis, Indiana

**STEPHEN PERKINS, MD**
Clinical Associate Professor, Department
of Otolaryngology–Head and Neck Surgery,
Indiana University School of Medicine; and
Meridian Plastic Surgeons and Medical Skin
Care, Indianapolis, Indiana

**KRISTA RODRIGUEZ-BRUNO, MD**
Resident, Department of Otolaryngology,
Head and Neck Surgery, University of
California, San Francisco, California

**JACOB D. STEIGER, MD**
Clinical Lecturer, Department of
Otolaryngology, Center for Facial Cosmetic
Surgery, University of Michigan, Livonia,
Michigan

**RAVI S. SWAMY, MD, MPH**
Division of Facial Plastic and Reconstructive
Surgery, Stanford University School of
Medicine, Stanford, California

**JONATHAN M. SYKES, MD, FACS**
Professor and Director, Facial Plastic and
Reconstructive Surgery, Department of
Otolaryngology, University of California,
Davis, Sacramento

**DEAN M. TORIUMI, MD**
Professor, Department of Otolaryngology–
Head and Neck Surgery, University of Illinois,
Chicago, Illinois

**DEBORAH WATSON, MD, FACS**
Associate Professor and Residency Program
Director, Division of Otolaryngology-Head
and Neck Surgery; Director, Facial Plastic
and Reconstructive Surgery, UCSD School
of Medicine, San Diego, California

# Contents

> The business of rhinoplasty has undergone changes in keeping with increased competitive pressures locally, nationally, and internationally. Patient demands and progress in the field have abolished the "cookie-cutter" nose, with patients now requesting extensive discussions and predictions with computer photoimaging. The R-Factor Question and The D.O.S. Conversation are effective tools in rhinoplasty consultations. These tools provide patients with the clarity of what surgery can do for their lives and help patients overcome the fear produced by the overwhelming amount of information available. By helping our patients achieve the next level of success in their lives, we guarantee ourselves a busy practice filled with happy patients. The rhinoplasty consultation is the key to beginning this relationship of success.

> The perioperative period can be anxiety provoking for rhinoplasty patients. Patients rely on the skill and confidence of the surgeon to attain optimal results. Having an established strategy for the preoperative, anesthetic, and postoperative care of this patient population is critical to achieving a successful outcome and to ensuring a positive experience for the patient. Establishing a sincere rapport in the preoperative period and being able to properly address patient concerns regarding anesthesia helps patients develop a positive frame of mind and aids in their recovery. This presentation reviews important elements of the preoperative, anesthetic, and postoperative care of rhinoplasty patients and provides insight to making the experience a positive one for the patient and the surgeon.

> Profile refinement is one of the most common reasons patients seek consultation for rhinoplasty. Emphasis on creating a natural-appearing nasal dorsum demands a methodic nasal and facial analysis. Areas of dorsal excess and deficiency are identified, quantitated, and considered when determining surgical goals. The radix is an essential component of the profile and is carefully assessed from the standpoint of projection and position. Height and contour are evaluated at the radix, rhinion, and nasal tip. Each component of the dorsal profile is individually classified as overprojected, underprojected, or of appropriate height. Case studies demonstrate the necessary surgical steps to create a more balanced profile.

> In rhinoplasty, the nasal tip remains the most challenging anatomic region to diag-
> nose and treat. This article presents a new concept, the M-arch model, to better un-
> derstand the functional and aesthetic anatomy of the tip. This M-arch can be
> lengthened or shortened, or left as is, to establish the basis of ideal nasal length, pro-
> jection, and rotation. Additional suture, incisional, excisional, and grafting maneu-
> vers can be performed in a graduated fashion to further refine the M-arch,
> including the lobule and soft tissue of the nasal base. A full description of the
> M-arch model and its application is presented, and representative results are
> illustrated.

> Suture modification techniques have long served as reliable methods to surgically
> improve nasal tip contour by allowing control of width, projection, and rotation dur-
> ing rhinoplasty. Tip abnormalities characterized by a wide or broad shape are par-
> ticularly amenable to such techniques. In the senior author's hands (SWP), the
> endonasal double-dome tip-sculpting technique has become a workhorse for the
> correction of the wide tip complex. When combined with additional techniques,
> the double-dome technique allows for the correction of various abnormalities falling
> under the umbrella of a broad tip (ie, boxy, bifid, bulbous, trapezoid, amorphous),
> while still adhering to the tenets of modern rhinoplasty philosophy. The authors pres-
> ent a paradigm for surgical planning, along with a series of case studies highlighting
> the capabilities of various suture techniques performed with the endonasal
> approach.

> The authors introduce the concept of favorable shadowing of the nasal tip surface.
> Contouring the nasal tip is an advanced concept in rhinoplasty. Several tip altering
> techniques exist, but proper selection of an appropriate technique or combination of
> techniques first requires understanding of the impact of manipulating underlying tip
> structure on nasal surface topography. Frequently, maneuvers that narrow the
> domes, inappropriately create a pinched or unnatural-appearing nasal tip. Many
> of these tip-narrowing techniques act to lower the caudal margin of the lateral crura
> below the cephalic margin and decrease support along the junction between the tip
> and alar lobule. The nasal tip skin can then collapse on this structure, creating a vis-
> ible line of demarcation between the tip and alar lobule. Patients will describe their
> operated nasal tip as having the appearance of a round ball or bulbous tip, even
> thought their nasal tip may be narrow. This pinched appearance is due to the shad-
> owing that isolates the nasal tip, creating a bulbous or pinched look to the nasal tip.
> Maneuvers such as dome sutures, lateral crural strut grafts, repositioning of the lat-
> eral crura, and alar rim grafts can create a favorable tip structure to support the un-
> derlying skin envelope. Using the methods described will enable the surgeon to
> focus less on narrowing the nasal tip and more on creating favorable shadowing
> of the nasal tip.

Advances in grafting techniques have provided the basis for a paradigm shift in rhinoplasty in which purely reductive techniques have been largely supplanted by structurally sound framework surgery. Proficiency with autologous cartilage grafting allows the rhinoplasty surgeon to achieve superior nasal definition and durable aesthetic outcomes by building a stable nasal framework that resists the contractile forces of healing responsible for delayed nasal airway compromise and aesthetic distortion. Cartilage grafts may be used to reposition, augment, or reconstitute nasal structure after cartilaginous resection and recontouring. The authors present various grafting techniques that are reliably used to sculpt the nasal framework in rhinoplasty, with emphasis on the relevant anatomy, nomenclature, and clinical indications for each approach. Judicious use of these methods results in predictable rhinoplasty outcomes with enhanced aesthetics and function.

The complete rhinoplasty surgeon must possess an understanding of functional nasal airway obstruction. An increasingly sophisticated grasp of the pathophysiology of fixed nasal obstruction has led surgeons to develop and refine surgical techniques aimed toward alleviating nasal valve insufficiency. This article reviews an assortment of techniques within nasal valve surgery, highlighting the underlying pathophysiology, anatomy, and technical considerations.

Many surgical approaches and techniques to repair cleft nasal deformities have been described. Because the presenting patient with a congenital deformity is young, the surgical plan must account for patient growth and surgical scarring. The surgeon should understand the pathophysiology of the deformity and have a systematic surgical plan. This article describes the classic nasal abnormalities associated with clefting of the lip, and outlines surgical techniques and timing used to minimize these deformities.

The surgical maneuvers employed in aesthetic rhinoplasty can result in unforeseen structural complications that lead to an unsatisfied patient. Many of these problems arise years after the primary surgery and include both aesthetic and functional losses. Contemporary rhinoplasty should always be designed with long-term perspective and an eye on possible untoward outcomes. This article discusses the anatomic and physiologic basis of rhinoplasty complications with a focus on primary rhinoplasty principles that will prevent their formation.

Deborah Watson

Tissue engineering is a rapidly evolving field of research, and its impact on clinical health care solutions can be profound. It offers a unique opportunity to bridge the gap between basic science and the application of a tissue-engineered cartilage product for patients undergoing primary and revision rhinoplasty. Autologous tissue-engineered septal cartilage can be fabricated from a small sample of septal cartilage taken from a patient. This tissue-engineered product would eventually provide the surgeon with adequate grafting material with which to complete a rhinoplasty or nasal reconstructive case without the known limitations of tissue availability and tissue quantity. An update on this technology is presented as it relates to our field.

# Facial Plastic Surgery Clinics of North America

**THE CLINICS ARE NOW AVAILABLE ONLINE!**

Access your subscription at:
**www.theclinics.com**

# Preface

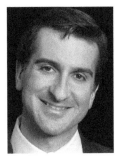

Minas Constantinides, MD, FACS
*Guest Editor*

Rhinoplasty has evolved more quickly over the past 10 years than in any other time of the past 100 years. Breakthrough to this evolution has been the open technique, in which the entire structure of the nose can be inspected accurately and favorably distorted to effect maximal cosmetic and functional change. Today, the operated-on nose can be stronger and more stable than the virgin nose. Minimal excisions of cartilage, coupled with adding cartilaginous support from the septum, ear, and rib, have permitted unprecedented change, truly allowing plasticity in the result.

The feuds among egos of the past, trading progress in knowledge for divided camps of thought, have been largely supplanted by collegial exchanges of information among disciples of rhinoplasty. It is common today to see plastic surgeons and facial plastic surgeons put aside differences to share a common stage, furthering exchange of knowledge at unprecedented rates.

Despite all the knowledge that experience has given the field, there is still much to learn. The challenge is never to be complacent and content with our results but to continue being self-critical and ever examining our thinking and skills. Technologic advances promise amazing horizons of new tissue engineering techniques, further expanding what we are able to achieve surgically.

In this issue are assembled the thoughts of some of the best minds in rhinoplasty today. Some are widely recognized as leaders in the field, whereas others represent the emerging next generation that should break new ground in the future. All have already made a tremendous contribution to our field. I hope you enjoy what they have to teach.

Minas Constantinides, MD, FACS
Department of Otolaryngology–Head and Neck Surgery
New York University School of Medicine
530 First Avenue, Suite 7U
New York, NY 10016

E-mail address:
minas.constantinides@med.nyu.edu

Facial Plast Surg Clin N Am 17 (2009) xi
doi:10.1016/j.fsc.2008.10.003

# The Rhinoplasty Consultation and the Business of Rhinoplasty

Minas Constantinides, MD, FACS

**KEYWORDS**

- Rhinoplasty • Consultation • The R-factor question
- The D.O.S. conversation • Body dysmorphic disorder

With the explosion of information that the Internet has brought, the marketplace in rhinoplasty has become more global. The outsourcing to Bangalore, India, of computer help and banking customer service has transformed those industries.[1] Similarly, our own competitors are no longer simply the surgeon down the block, but the surgeon across the ocean. The best-known international plastic surgery center has long been in Rio de Janeiro, Brazil, where Dr. Ivo Pitanguy has long attracted international patients to his private island for surgery and posh recovery. Mexico has been a destination for HIV-infected patients seeking non–FDA-approved fillers for their facial lipoatrophy. Now, Mexican centers are expanding into facelifting and rhinoplasty. Colombian surgeons are fashioning English Web sites to compete directly for United States consumers. In Turkey, the crossroads between Europe, Asia, and the Arabic world, surgeons are building hospitals on the Mediterranean where even middle class patients can have surgery and recover more economically than with similar surgery in London or New York. Korea is the Mecca for Asian blepharoplasty, to which even United States–born Asians are flying for their surgery. These international plastic surgery destinations are exploding in number and attracting patients worldwide. How, then, does the individual rhinoplasty surgeon remain competitive with so many more competitors, both local and international?

The Internet has vastly increased the amount of information available to the patient about rhinoplasty; however, this unfiltered information from doctors' sites, patients' blogs, chat rooms, and third-party sites is overwhelming, confusing, and frustrating. Many chat-room participants are those who have been unhappy with their rhinoplasty and are looking to make a connection with others who share their feelings of frustration and abandonment. This confusion and frustration can be paralyzing for new and revision patients looking for reliable information.

Providers often add to the confusion. Self-serving Web sites replete with misleading information about an operation "invented" by the "expert" host surgeon try to capture unwitting patients who do not possess the knowledge to filter truth from falsehoods. When fear and uncertainty are the main outcomes of overwhelming information, making a positive decision for surgery becomes impossible.

Consider, on the other hand, the opportunity. If we can act as effective filters of information by clarifying and simplifying it, imagine the relief we can offer our patients. This clarity will provide such value to confused and frustrated patients that they will be able to overcome the fears that this information creates and allow them to make informed surgical decisions.

What can we do as surgeons to convince new patients to stay local for their surgeries? First, let us explore what does not work.

## SCARE TACTICS

Scare tactics may seem like a great way to make patients see how much better you are than your competitor. A typical scare tactic would be, "If you go next door (or around the world) to the

Facial Plast Surg Clin N Am 17 (2009) 1–5
doi:10.1016/j.fsc.2008.09.005

cheaper, less experienced surgeon, you will have a higher risk of complications, have poor results, and not be happy. So, use me instead."

Scare tactics do not work. People choose their physician on the basis of feelings of safety and security. People choose a product or service because it gives them pleasure or enhances their potential. Scare tactics play to people's fears, not their hopes; create negative feelings about the messenger; and do nothing to actualize the person.

## COMMODITY THINKING

Commodity thinking is a trap that the young practitioner easily falls into. It involves lowering price to capture more market share (more patients). The practitioner might say, "I am not only a board-certified surgeon but I also have the best price in town. Why pay more for the same surgery?" If this sounds like a used-car salesman, then that is exactly how the patient will interpret it.

Commodities are things we buy and sell. Large companies, like Coca-Cola, Dell, and Microsoft, succeed by improving their production efficiencies so that they can lower their products' prices, undercutting the competition while improving their profits. These companies are successful until their competitors lower their own prices even more.

Rhinoplasty surgeons and other cosmetic service providers are not such large companies with a dominant market share. We provide value-added services that are quality driven and innovative; we are able to diversify quickly. The key is to identify the value that our patients derive from our services. If we can help our patients understand complex information and fulfill their future vision of themselves, then the value we can provide is tremendous. This simple idea—that our goal is to help enhance our patients' lives by helping them actualize their visions of themselves—is priceless.

Consider this in your own life. If someone could help you figure out what you want to achieve in your life, both personally and professionally, and then help you successfully achieve that vision, what would you pay? For many, the answer is, "I would pay almost anything."

When we, as surgeons, help our patients see their future potential and then help them achieve a part of that vision, we become indispensable instruments of positive change in their lives. We are not only promising a great rhinoplasty but are also promising to help them achieve their future vision of themselves in which rhinoplasty plays an important part (if it did not, they would not be seeing us in consultation). When we stop thinking of ourselves are surgeons and start thinking of

ourselves as transformers of lives through surgery—helping our patients achieve the next level of success in their lives—we guarantee ourselves a busy practice filled with happy patients. The rhinoplasty consultation is the key to beginning this relationship of success.

## THE RHINOPLASTY CONSULTATION

A patient sits in your reception area waiting to meet with you. He looks like any other patient. Because he is coming for essentially the same discussion ("What can you do for my nose"), you assume his expectations, fears, and concerns are the same as everyone else's. Indeed, the further he is from you in age, the more you assume about who he is and what he wants. You ask friendly questions about his job, his family, and how long he has been in the area, and your brain fills in the blanks to imagine his life around his rhinoplasty request. You then get to the business of discussing his nose, and let him know what he can expect with you as his surgeon.

There are many problems with this consultation model. First, it is boring for the surgeon. After having many consultations with essentially the same beginning and ending, they feel routine. This feeling is something the patient interprets as a rushed or superficial consultation that is not gratifying for him or for you. Second, and more important, the assumptions you make to fill in the gaps of information are almost invariably wrong. The very fabric of the life a 20- or 30-year-old today is very different than the one you lived. Relationships are different, interactions are different, communication is different.

The best approach is to not have preconceived ideas about anything and to let the patient drive the interaction completely. This approach can be achieved by asking unstructured or open-ended questions to get as much information about the patient's life and to determine how it fits into his desire for rhinoplasty. Below, I outline my structured sequence of obtaining this information from patients. I have adapted this sequence from "The Strategic Coach Program," created by Dan Sullivan, which coaches entrepreneurs from many different businesses.[2]

## THE R-FACTOR QUESTION

As soon as a patient enters my office, I ask them how they found out about me. I track these answers to determine the efficacy of my various referral sources. The next question I ask is, "What do you want to talk about today?" The answer, for our purposes here, is some variation of "My nose." The third thing I ask is a question adapted from The R-Factor Question[†] ("R" stands for relationship):

*"If we were to meet here in one year, looking back over that year, what would have had to have happened, both personally and professionally, for you to be satisfied with your progress in your life?"*

The R-Factor Question immediately builds a relationship of trust between the physician and patient. It helps to clarify for the patient his goals for the coming year, and frames the surgery among those goals. It directly ties his life goals with what you have to offer him as his surgeon. He is no longer shopping for a commodity (rhinoplasty), but is being offered a relationship of growth leading to fulfilling his life goals. This relationship, when established, is long lasting and nearly impossible to break.

As the surgeon interviewer, it is very tempting to interrupt with positive comments about what you can offer the patient. Interrupting, however, is like telling the patient that you have heard enough and now want to talk about yourself. You must overcome the delusion that the patient wants to hear about you at this point. The patient wants to talk about himself, his goals, and his dreams. You must give him the chance to do so without adding your editorials and superlatives. There will be time for that later. It is also important to carefully record his answers. This will allow you to accurately refer to them later in the consultation and during subsequent visits.

Here are some actual answers from patients:

*"I am happy with life as it is."*
*"I want to be able to enjoy life more."*
*"I want to look better."*
*"I want to lose some weight."*
*"I want to be settled in new job."*
*"My wedding will be over."*
*"I will feel less self-conscious."*
*"I want to wake up every morning and not have to think about my nose."*

Most answers have little to do with rhinoplasty. It is the surgeon's job to show how rhinoplasty can fit into these goals.

At times, when I ask The R-Factor Question, the patient is confused. He is used to being hurried into a consultation room, spending 5 minutes speaking with the doctor, being given a plan, and then being asked to schedule surgery. My consultations last between 30 and 60 minutes, depending on the complexity of the patient's fears and on any previous experiences with surgery. If a patient hesitates or answers only the question with regard to surgical outcome, I ask them to tell me about their other personal hopes and goals for the next year. If the patient is still confused, I explain that I want to understand how surgery will fit into their lives and want to know something more about that. Generally, this explanation is sufficient for a patient to feel confident enough to answer fully.

Sometimes a patient refuses to answer The R-Factor Question. In those rare cases, I politely explain that I am not the right surgeon for them. This patient does not want a relationship of growth with me. He sees me as a commodity, one that he can buy for himself at the right price (which he will invariably haggle about). He is not someone I want in my practice.

## THE D.O.S. CONVERSATION

After the R-Factor Question is answered and the answer is recorded, The D.O.S. Conversation[1] begins. This discussion is a continuation of The R-Factor Question and includes the dangers, opportunities, and strengths (D.O.S.) that apply to rhinoplasty for that specific patient.

### *Dangers*

The next question is about the dangers the patient sees pertaining to achieving his goals for the next year, in particular regarding rhinoplasty. I ask, "When thinking about rhinoplasty, what do you worry about?" Everyone worries about something pertaining to any important decision. By discussing the worries early and resolving them, you allow a patient to focus on the positive rather than the negative. Any unresolved worry, compounded by the confusion of all the unfiltered information available on the Internet, paralyzes a patient's ability to proceed with rhinoplasty. By resolving the worry early in the encounter, the patient can focus on the positive and proceed with scheduling surgery. Here are some answers to the danger question:

*"A 'done' look": "Michael Jackson," "Kenny Rogers," "Joan Rivers."*
*"Not waking up from anesthesia."*
*"A result that is not what I want."*
*"Trouble breathing after surgery."*
*"I have read…online, and wonder…."*

---

[†]The R-Factor Question, D.O.S., and The D.O.S. Conversation are registered trademarks and copyrighted works owned by The Strategic Coach, Inc. All rights reserved. Used with written permission. www.strategiccoach.com.

*"Recovery time, and finding time in my schedule to do this."*

*"Cost."*

By helping the patient overcome the dangers he faces, you provide important leadership, allowing him to see how he can attain his goals in rhinoplasty despite his fears.

## Opportunities

Discussing fears is the only negative conversation you will have with the patient. After this negative discussion, a positive one is important to bring up the patient's excitement about his potential after surgery. This positive discussion is achieved through the opportunities question:

*"Now pretend that one year has passed, and you have had successful rhinoplasty. What will that do for you?"*

This question allows the patient to envision himself on the other side of surgery and recovery. How will his life look then? How will it be different than it is now? Remarkably, many patients have not thought about this. They are so focused and worried about the surgery that they have not articulated to themselves all the benefits that surgery will give them. The following are some responses:

*"I won't have to wake up every morning and see this nose."*

*"I will be more competitive in my professional life."*

*"I've been thinking of surgery for a long time. I'll be able to move on in my life."*

*"I'll feel more self-confident."*

*"I won't have to think about my nose every time I meet someone new."*

## Strengths

After discussing opportunities, it is helpful to frame the discussion around the strengths that the patient already has. In this way, he sees how the new opportunities that rhinoplasty will give him will reinforce and build on his current strengths, creating new strengths to apply in his life. If a patient's current strengths have not been discussed during earlier parts of the conversation, they can be discussed now: "What are your personal strengths, and how will surgery build on them?" The following are some responses:

*"I am already a pretty confident person, but this will make me more so."*

*"I'll be able to breathe better, so I can exercise better."*

*"I'll look better for my age."*

The R-Factor Question and The D.O.S. Conversation are powerful tools that produce meaningful insights on a number of levels. From the patient's perspective, the interaction has focused him on his future vision of himself and put surgery into the context of his life. By just listening and encouraging an open-ended conversation, the surgeon is framed as the architect of the patient's further personal growth. Most of our patients are successful in their lives already. Patients are looking for that thing that will make them better and help them reach their next level of personal growth. In a developed, modern society, after basic needs are met and people are financially secure, personal growth becomes a primary focus. For proof, merely look at the boom in personal trainers, health clubs, yoga classes, and holistic living. This concept derives from the five levels of Maslow's pyramid.[3] These levels, from bottom to top, are physiologic (survival), safety, love/belonging, esteem (achievement), and self-actualization. Surgery, because of its power to produce dramatic change in a short time, is very compelling.

From the surgeon's perspective, The D.O.S. Conversation provides powerful insight into the true motivation for surgery. When we understand why our patients want surgery (and not just what they want done), we can more easily help them to overcome their fears and see the value we can bring to their lives. Indeed, the single most important outcome of The D.O.S. Conversation is to show patients the value we can bring to them. Effective surgery is valuable. But to help a patient elevate himself to the next level he sees for himself in his life is much more valuable. This is the competitive edge we need to succeed in this increasingly competitive world.

The D.O.S. Conversation is also excellent for uncovering body dysmorphic disorder and patients who are not good candidates for surgery. For example, if teenaged patients cannot have a meaningful conversation about their future, I believe that they are not good candidates for surgery and politely suggest that they return when they are older.

Establishing a relationship with our patients is crucial before agreeing to surgery. When I was younger in my practice, I had one of my best surgical outcomes in a patient who was my most dissatisfied to date. This patient, a man from London, found me on the Internet and began an e-mail discussion with me about revising his nose. Even though he had many questions, I diligently answered them, faithfully reviewing the poor-quality photos that he sent to me. Finally, we agreed to surgery. He arrived the day before the scheduled surgery, 2 hours after my office was supposed to close, having chosen a flight that was convenient only to him. I performed photoimaging for him, and after we agreed on a plan, I performed surgery. His recovery was uneventful surgically, but he was unhappy from the first day after surgery. He could not be consoled that what he was seeing was swelling. After surgery, he returned to London and focused on how devastated his nose looked to him. Objectively, the result was excellent, but he saw only problems. Finally, we agreed that our best course was to part ways, and I refunded his money after he signed a legal release (advice from my malpractice attorneys).

What went wrong? Although one could argue that he had body dysmorphic disorder and should never have had surgery (probably true), I believe the main error was not having a relationship of growth with the patient. I fell into what I have coined "the expert complex": "Since I am one of the few real expert rhinoplasty surgeons, if I do not help this poor patient, he will be forced to go elsewhere and seek inferior help from an inferior surgeon, with inferior or damaging results." Strangely, as I have become more experienced in rhinoplasty, I no longer believe this. Now, my most important criterion is not the nose that I am facing but the relationship that I can have with the patient behind the nose.

Many other important aspects of the rhinoplasty consultation are covered by other contributors in this issue. There are many ways to build a strong relationship with patients. The R-Factor Question and The D.O.S. Conversation are tools that I have found effective in my practice. The clarity they provide to patients of what surgery can do for their lives makes them compelling and powerful. They help patients overcome the fear produced by the overwhelming amount of information available today and lead to effectivelife-changing surgery.

## REFERENCES

1. Friedman TL. The world is flat: a brief history of the twenty-first century. New York: Farrar, Struas & Giroux; 2005.
2. Sullivan D. The Strategic Coach, Inc. 33 Fraser Ave., Ste. 201, Toronto, Ontario, Canada.
3. Sullivan D. The global thinker. Toronto: The Strategic Coach, Inc.; 2008.

# Preoperative, Anesthetic, and Postoperative Care for Rhinoplasty Patients

Ravi S. Swamy, MD, MPH, Sam P. Most, MD*

KEYWORDS

- Rhinoplasty • Preoperative care
- Anesthetic care • Postoperative care

## PREOPERATIVE CARE

An educated patient is more likely to have a positive perioperative experience. After the initial consultation and when the surgical plan is complete, rhinoplasty patients in the authors' care undergo a structured preoperative visit to ensure that all concerns are addressed, all questions are answered, and the patient and the surgeon have a shared understanding of the goals of the surgery. This visit takes place 1 week before the scheduled surgery date.

All patients fill out a preoperative questionnaire detailing their past medical, surgical, and anesthetic history, including a list of current medications. Patients who are on aspirin or other medications that may disturb normal platelet function were told at earlier visits (in collaboration with their prescribing doctors) that these medications should be stopped 2 weeks before the surgery date. Patients who smoke are asked to avoid smoking and using other nicotine-containing products for 4 weeks before surgery because their effects on wound healing is well documented.[1]

After the patient completes the questionnaire, the surgeon reviews the responses and performs a thorough physical examination, including auscultation of the heart and lungs. After addressing all potential issues concerning the patient's general health and well-being, the surgeon can now focus on the nasal analysis and evaluation.

Although nasal evaluation is assessed at the initial visit, it is important to review pertinent findings and get reacquainted with the patient's anatomy before surgery. The primary concerns of the patient and what he or she hopes to achieve through surgery must be paramount. After the surgeon iterates and validates these concerns, analysis should begin broadly. After assessing the symmetry and proportions of the nose to the face, it is important to evaluate the thickness, integrity, and mobility of the skin–soft tissue envelope in relation to the underlying nasal structures, because it dictates what can be accomplished intraoperatively.[2] Another critical factor in assessing the patient is to determine through careful palpation the inherent strength and support of the nasal tip. A patient who has weak tip support will not tolerate extensive removal of cartilage but may require the addition of supportive grafts and struts to improve the tip's stability and support. Patients who have strong tip support can tolerate reduction maneuvers that improve refinement. The size, shape, attitude, and resilience of the alar cartilages can be estimated by palpation or ballottement of the lateral crus between two fingers surrounding its cephalic and caudal margins. During this assessment, the surgeon makes the all-important decision about whether to enhance, reduce, or carefully preserve the tip projection that exists preoperatively.[3]

Division of Facial Plastic and Reconstructive Surgery, Stanford University School of Medicine, 801 Welch Road, Stanford, CA 94305, USA
* Corresponding author.
*E-mail address:* smost@ohns.stanford.edu (S.P. Most).

Facial Plast Surg Clin N Am 17 (2009) 7–13
doi:10.1016/j.fsc.2008.09.006

Just as it is important to recognize the main aesthetic concerns of the patient, it is important for the surgeon to highlight and point out the more subtle findings. If unaddressed, the scrutinizing patient may notice these postoperatively, negating an otherwise positive outcome.[4]

Even in cases of cosmetic rhinoplasty, careful evaluation and documentation of the nasal airway and discussion of symptoms of nasal obstruction are addressed in detail. Many cosmetic patients may have underlying symptoms of nasal obstruction that go undiagnosed and may become a source of complaint postoperatively.[4] On occasion, the use of rigid or flexible endoscopes may yield useful information that could affect surgical planning.[5]

Previous to the preoperative visit, standardized digital photographs from the frontal, base, lateral, and oblique views are taken. These images are also computer enhanced to simulate surgical goals. They are excellent communication tools, and satisfaction with cosmetic surgery after computer imaging has been documented to be higher than in those patients who did not receive imaging.[6] Computer imaging not only facilitates discussion about specific goals of the procedure but it also helps to uncover any potential unrealistic expectations of the patient.[7] It must be stressed to the patient that the images represent a means to facilitate discussion and to improve their education of what can and cannot be accomplished. It is the surgeon's responsibility to temper the patient's desires to realistic goals. Every effort is made to reproduce these images, which are used intraoperatively. Images are displayed in the operating suite, and an attempt is made to match the enhanced images to the patient on the table. A study by Agarwal and colleagues[7] illustrated that computer imaging for rhinoplasty patients portrays a realistic picture of actual postoperative results; however, they state that it is important for the surgeon to be able to use this modality with discretion because the computer images should be restricted to the confines of the surgeon's abilities.

While reviewing the photographic images, it is critical to review the goals of surgery and ensure that the issues the patient would like addressed have not changed. During the preoperative evaluation, the surgeon must possess a mental image of the potential outcome and the surgical limitations inherent in every individual case. In essence, the operation is rehearsed as the preoperative evaluation proceeds.[4]

After the surgical goals are reviewed and the plan is mutually understood between the patient and the surgeon, the patient is given a standardized medical procedure informed consent form and a rhinoplasty-specific consent form outlining the specific skin incisions that will be used. The authors hand-write the specifics of the procedure and repeat the goals of the surgery. The patient is encouraged to ask questions, and every effort is made to explain the risks, benefits, and alternatives using terminology that the patient can easily comprehend. Possible complications are also discussed. Complications rates from rhinoplasty vary between 10% and 15%.[4] Complications can be categorized as aesthetic or functional in nature. A candid discussion with the patient regarding the possibility of a complication is imperative, with the acknowledgment that every effort will be made to correct the complication if it occurs (most complications are correctable).[8] The patient should also be made aware of the temporary swelling, ecchymosis, and nasal obstruction in the immediate postoperative period. An intimate knowledge of the patient's unique nasal anatomy and accurate preoperative analysis are crucial to achieving the desired long-term postoperative result and to avoiding preventable complications.

After completing the informed consent process, patients are given postoperative prescriptions in advance. Typically, patients are placed on narcotic medications for pain and prophylactic antibiotic for 5 days. The authors do not give their patients a steroid taper. Studies have shown that postoperative steroids are not effective in reducing postoperative edema and subject patients to undue risk.[9–11] Preoperative orders in anticipation of surgery are also completed at this visit. There is a standardized work-up of ancillary testing for patients undergoing a procedure under general anesthesia (**Table 1**). Patients meet with the clinical nurse to discuss the details of the operative day, including the time and location of the surgery, perioperative diet, and final costs of the procedure.

## ANESTHETIC CARE

All patients undergoing rhinoplasty have their surgery at an accredited ambulatory surgery center and are given the opportunity to meet the anesthesiologist preoperatively. All issues regarding the anesthesia are answered, and a thorough history and physical examination is performed. Although this procedure may be repetitive, it allows the anesthesiologist to formulate an appropriate plan for anesthesia well ahead of the actual surgery date. In addition, most patients gain comfort in knowing that all members of the surgical team share a similar goal of achieving a good outcome while placing priority on their safety and well-being throughout this process.

**Table 1**
**Ancillary test recommendations for patients scheduled for surgical procedures under general anesthesia**

| Age (y) | Male Patients | Female Patients |
| --- | --- | --- |
| <40 | None | Pregnancy test |
| 40–49 | ECG | Pregnancy test, hematocrit |
| 50–64 | ECG | Hematocrit, ECG |
| 65–74 | ECG, hematocrit, blood urea nitrogen, glucose | Hematocrit, ECG, blood urea nitrogen, glucose |
| >75 | ECG, hematocrit, blood urea nitrogen, glucose, chest radiograph | Hematocrit, ECG, blood urea nitrogen glucose, chest radiograph |

*Data from* Feisher LA, Johns RA, Savarese JJ, et al. Miller's anesthesia. 6th edition. London: Churchill Livingstone; 2005, p. 2594.

It has been well documented that rhinoplasty can be performed with local anesthesia and intravenous sedation or with general anesthesia.[12] The risks of intravenous sedation and general anesthesia are well known; therefore, the surgeon and anesthesia personnel should do what they are most comfortable executing, keeping patient safety as the principal concern.[13]

The authors advocate an intravenous-only general anesthesia using a laryngeal mask for their rhinoplasty patients. General anesthesia in the hands of well-trained anesthetists using advanced monitoring and pharmacologic techniques on a healthy patient is safe and effective. With general anesthesia, tighter blood pressure control can be achieved, thereby minimizing intraoperative bleeding. The authors also believe that the laryngeal mask significantly reduces the risk of aspiration in nasal surgery. Patients are comfortably and fully asleep, allowing the surgeon to focus full attention on the operation without the distraction of inadvertent patient movement and elimination of the seesaw effect of intravenous sedation.[14]

### The Authors' Protocol

The patient is asked to arrive 2 hours before the scheduled time of surgery and is met by the clinical nurse who already has an established rapport with the patient. After changing into a surgical gown, the patient meets again with the anesthesiologist to go over the plan of anesthesia in the preoperative holding area. The patient is also given three doses of 0.05% oxymetazoline nasal spray to each nostril spaced 10 minutes apart to help with decongestion and vasoconstriction. The surgeon arrives to greet the patent and reviews the surgical plan one last time. Every effort is made to keep the atmosphere tranquil to reduce patient anxiety.

The anesthesiologist injects a small amount of 2% lidocaine diluted 1:1 with sodium bicarbonate to reduce the acidity of the lidocaine, and places an intravenous line. The anesthesiologist then administers 2 mg of midazolam for anxiolytic purposes and escorts the patient to the operating suite. The operating room is kept quiet, and conversation by the staff is kept to an absolute minimum.

After properly positioning the patient on the table and ensuring his or her comfort, preoxygenation by way of facemask begins. For induction, the patient is given 25 μg of fentanyl and 200 mg of propofol. If the patient has a history of severe nausea and vomiting associated with anesthesia, 4 mg of odansetron is also given. An $\alpha_2$-adrenergic agonist drug such as clonidine may also be infused because it can reduce anesthetic and analgesic dosage requirements and produce sedation and anxiolysis while also decreasing the heart rate and blood pressure during anesthesia; however, residual postoperative sedation may be a problem for elderly outpatients.[14] After the patient is induced, a short-acting muscle relaxant such as cisatracurium is given if the patient is expected to be intubated with an endotracheal tube. As mentioned earlier, the authors prefer the use of laryngeal mask airway (LMA). Tracheal intubation causes a high incidence of postoperative airway-related complaints, including sore throat, croup, and hoarseness. One study showed that the incidence of postoperative sore throat after ambulatory surgery was 18% with an LMA versus 45% with a tracheal tube.[15] Most outpatients undergoing superficial procedures under general anesthesia do not require tracheal intubation unless they are at high risk for aspiration.[16] Compared with tracheal intubation, insertion of the LMA causes minimal cardiovascular responses and is better tolerated at lighter levels of anesthesia.[17] The LMA also prevents the patient from swallowing blood during the procedure that could contribute to postoperative nausea and emesis. When endotracheal tubes are used, the authors place a throat pack to prevent blood from entering the esophageal inlet.

After securing the airway, the anesthesiologist gives the patient a prophylactic antibiotic such as 1 g of cefazolin, or 600 mg of clindamycin for patients who have penicillin allergies. Intravenous corticosteroids are routinely administered to reduce postoperative nausea and postoperative swelling.[9]

Prior to sterilely cleansing and draping the patient, it is important to properly prepare the nose for surgery. **Fig. 1** illustrates the tools used in the authors' typical preparation tray. The use of a sharp pair of Iris scissors allows the surgeon to cut the vibrissae for improved visualization of incisions. A 10-mL control syringe with a 1.50-in, 27-gauge needle is used to inject the local anesthetic. Local anesthetics produce sensory loss by blocking excitatory stimulation at the nerve endings and by inhibiting conduction in the peripheral nerve tissue, thereby reducing the amount of general anesthetic required.[15] Although there are many different forms of local anesthetics, the authors prefer 1% lidocaine with 1:100,000 epinephrine due to its efficacy, length of duration, and safety profile.[18] The maximum dose of lidocaine with epinephrine is 5 to 7 mg/kg, which can last up to 3.5 hours.[12] First, the septum is injected bilaterally in multiple sites beginning posteriorly. When completed properly, hydrodissection of mucoperichodrium can be achieved. Direct injection into the membranous septum is avoided to prevent a false hanging columella deformity. The pyriform aperture and nasal floor are also infiltrated. When turbinate reduction is planned, a small amount of local anesthetic can be injected into the inferior turbinates. For external

rhinoplasty approach, the columella is injected inferiorly and at its midpoint (**Fig. 2**A, B). The authors then insert the needle into the nasal tip and inject the dome, the medial crura, and supratip region (see **Fig. 2**C). The authors also inject the alar bases bilaterally to help with vasoconstriction of the lateral nasal branch of the facial artery (see **Fig. 2**D), followed by injection of the inferior edge of the lower lateral cartilages in preparation for the marginal incisions (**Fig. 3**A). Lastly, the nasal dorsum is injected subcutaneously through the vestibule immediately superficial to the nasal skeleton (see **Fig. 3**B). Less than 5 mL is used because any more can cause undo distortion. Cotton pledgets soaked in 0.05% oxymetazoline are placed bilaterally for continued decongestion and vasoconstriction. Although 4% cocaine can also be used, its cardiotoxic effects are well documented.[19–21] The patient's face is then prepared and draped in a sterile fashion. The authors prefer betadine scrub and paint. The first incision is not made until at least 10 minutes after injection of the local anesthetic so that the vasoconstrictive effects of the epinephrine can take place.

The patient ventilates spontaneously throughout the procedure. For maintenance, the anesthesiologist titrates a propofol drip and gives fentanyl as needed for analgesia. Blood pressure and heart rate are controlled with short-acting β-blockers such as esmolol. It is recommended to maintain the systolic blood pressure between 95 to 105 mm Hg to keep blood loss at a minimum, because clear visualization of the nasal anatomy is essential for a good outcome.

## POSTOPERATIVE CARE

After completion of the procedure, the dressings are placed and the recovery nurses are notified to expect the patient shortly. Communication between the surgeon and the anesthesiologist as to the end point of the operation is critical to ensure a smooth emergence. The oropharynx is gently suctioned with a Yankauer suction catheter. As the anesthetic is turned off and the patient becomes more aroused, the LMA is gently removed. The anesthesiologist is cognizant of the importance of awakening the patient quietly and smoothly and the avoidance of traumatic disruption of the surgical site. The surgeon is present for the emergence and ensures that the patient is safe before being moved to the recovery room. It can be reassuring for the patient to see the surgeon in this immediate postoperative period and hear words of encouragement regarding the surgery.

In the recovery room, attention should be on the patient's airway. Any mask placed on the patient

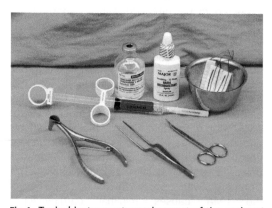

**Fig. 1.** Typical instruments used as part of the authors' preparation tray before the first incision, including Iris scissors, a nasal speculum, 1% lidocaine with 1:100,000 epinephrine, a 10-mL control syringe with 27-gauge needle, 0.05% oxymetazoline spray, and 0.5-in × 3-in cotton pledgets.

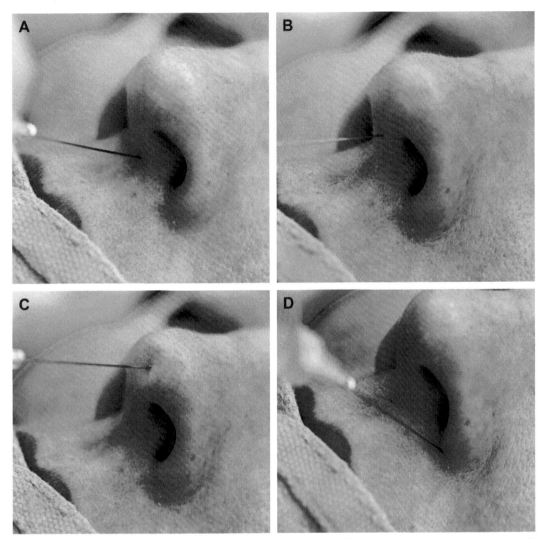

Fig. 2. Sites of injection of 1% lidocaine with 1:100,000 epinephrine. (*A, B*) Sites of injection on the columella. (*C*) Injection of the nasal tip. (*D*) Injection of the alar base.

for oxygenation should be done in such fashion as to not place pressure on the nose. The patient's head is elevated 30°, and cold compresses are gently placed over the eyes and nose. Care is taken to control postoperative pain, hypertension, and nausea as Valsalva can result in epistaxis or bleeding under the septal or nasal skin flaps. Patients who experience some epistaxis may have a folded 4 × 4 sponge placed under their nose that is held in place by a surgical mask cut into a thin rectangular piece.

After the patient is more alert and has stable vitals, the patient is transferred to a secondary recovery unit and allowed to change into his or her clothes. Patients are encouraged to wear buttoned shirts so that they do not have to pull clothes over their head and risk displacing the nasal splint.

Patients sit in a recliner at a 45° angle and are given clear liquids without carbonation if they are not nauseated. An intravenous line remains in place until discharge in the event that further antiemetic or pain medication is required.

During the recovery process, the patient's caregivers are given postoperative instructions and contact numbers for the staff and the surgeon. The clinical nurse goes over every detail of the instructions and ensures that all questions are answered. It is most important to address postoperative pain because it is frequently the most common issue. For those who are most concerned, the authors recommend taking the pain medication as prescribed every 6 hours for the first 24 hours, and then taking it as needed after that. Patients are also instructed to avoid blowing their nose and to

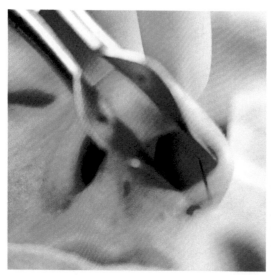
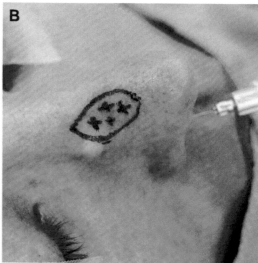

**Fig. 3.** (A) Injection of lidocaine along the lower lateral cartilages. (B) Transvestibular injections of the subcutaneous plane above the nasal skeleton. Markings of external contour are done before injection.

wipe the nose gently as needed. For minor postoperative bleeding, 0.05% oxymetazoline may be used sparingly for no more than 3 days. If the patient has continued bleeding, he or she should contact the surgeon immediately. The authors recommend that patients avoid nonsteroidal anti-inflammatory drugs because they affect platelet function and may lead to epistaxis. Patients are also told to avoid exerting themselves and to limit bending and lifting anything heavier than 10 lb. Restrictions are gradually lifted during the postoperative period as the patient recovers. Prior to discharge, the surgeon meets with the caregiver and the patient to go over the instructions and to address any concerns. Extra time spent in this critical period eases anxiety for the patient and the caregiver and assists in a quicker recovery. Patients are also given the time and date for their postoperative visit.

The surgeon contacts the patient on the evening of the surgery to reassure the patient and address any additional concerns. It is made clear to the patient that should any issue arise, the surgeon or a member of the staff is available at all times. The first postoperative visit takes place between postoperative day 5 and day 7. The nasal splint and columellar sutures are removed at this visit. Great care should be taken to gently remove the tape and splint over the nasal dorsum, which can be accomplished by first applying a generous amount of adhesive remover such as Detachol (Ferndale Laboratories, Ferndale, Michigan). After waiting a few minutes, blunt dissection of the nasal skin from the overlying splint using a cotton-tipped applicator avoids any disruption between the skin–soft tissue envelope and the underlying framework. Columellar sutures are then carefully removed. Patients will likely have a moderate amount of swelling and should be reminded that it can be almost a year before the final result is fully appreciated. Patients should avoid strenuous physical activity for 2 additional weeks and avoid heavy lifting (>10 lb). Patients can expect to resume full activity with no restrictions at 6 weeks after surgery.

In the authors' practice, patients are seen in the postoperative period at 1 week, 1 month, 3 months, 6 months, and 1 year. Frequent postoperative visits provide positive reinforcement to recovering patients and help to identify those who may not be satisfied or who have an unexpected outcome.

## SUMMARY

The challenges of rhinoplasty are substantial because every patient is unique and achieving success is multifaceted. A surgeon must not only possess a comprehensive set of surgical skills but also be able to effectively communicate with the patient and understand his or her concerns and desires. Although the surgery itself poses considerable challenges and can be a major source of anxiety, the implementation of an efficient perioperative strategy that can be consistently replicated can reduce trepidation and amplify success. This article describes the authors' approach to the preoperative, anesthetic, and postoperative care plan for patients undergoing rhinoplasty. There are many variations in perioperative planning, with no one correct strategy; however, all successful plans must foster open lines of communication and hold the patient's welfare in the highest regard.

## REFERENCES

1. Monfriecola G, Riccio G, Savarese C. The acute effect of smoking on cutaneous microcirculation blood flow in habitual smokers and nonsmokers. Dermatology 1998;197(2):115–8.
2. Tardy ME. Graduated sculpture refinement of the nasal tip. Facial Plast Surg Clin North Am 2004;12(1): 51–80.
3. Tardy ME. Rhinoplasty: the art and the science. Philadelphia: Saunders; 1997.
4. Becker DG, Becker SS. Reducing complications in rhinoplasty. Otolaryngol Clin North Am 2006;39(3):475–92.
5. Keck T, Leiacker R, Kühnemann S, et al. Video-endoscopy and digital image analysis of the nasal valve area. Eur Arch Otorhinolaryngol 2006;263(7):675–9.
6. Mühlbauer W, Holm C. Computer imaging and surgical reality in aesthetic rhinoplasty. Plast Reconstr Surg 2005;115(7):2098–104.
7. Agarwal A, Gracely E, Silver WE. Realistic expectations: to morph or not to morph? Plast Reconstr Surg 2007;119(4):1343–51.
8. Adamson PA, Litner JA. Psychologic aspects of revision rhinoplasty. Facial Plast Surg Clin North Am 2006;14(4):269–77.
9. Hoffmann DF, Cook TA, Quatela VC, et al. Steroids and rhinoplasty. A double-blind study. Arch Otolaryngol Head Neck Surg 1991;117(9):990–3.
10. Kara CO, Gökalan I. Effects of single-dose steroid usage on edema, ecchymosis, and intraoperative bleeding in rhinoplasty. Plast Reconstr Surg 1999;104(7):2213–8.
11. Kargi E, Hoşnuter M, Babucçu O, et al. Effect of steroids on edema, ecchymosis, and intraoperative bleeding in rhinoplasty. Ann Plast Surg 2003;51(6): 570–4.
12. Feisher LA, Johns RA, Savarese JJ, et al. Miller's anesthesia. 6th edition. London: Churchill Livingstone; 2005.
13. Ullmann Y, Levy Y, Isserles S, et al. Anesthesia for facial surgery. Aesthetic Plast Surg 1999;23(4): 296–7.
14. Hoefflin SM, Bornstein JB, Gordon M. General anesthesia in an office-based plastic surgical facility: a report on more than 23,000 consecutive office-based procedures under general anesthesia with no significant anesthetic complications. Plast Reconstr Surg 2001;107(1):243–51.
15. Higgins PP, Chung F, Mezei G. Postoperative sore throat after ambulatory surgery. Br J Anaesth 2002; 88(4):582–4.
16. Joshi GP, Inagaki Y, White PF. Use of the laryngeal mask airway as an alternative to the tracheal tube during ambulatory anesthesia. Anesth Analg 1997; 85(3):573–7.
17. Wat LI, Brimacombe JR, White PF. Use of the laryngeal mask airway in the ambulatory setting. J Clin Anesth 1998;10(5):386–8.
18. Cheney ML. Facial surgery: plastic and reconstructive. Baltimore: Williams & Wilkins; 1997.
19. Delilkan AE. Cocaine and adrenaline. Anaesth Intensive Care 1987;15(4):466–7.
20. Delilkan AE, Gnanapragasam A. Topical cocaine/adrenaline combination in intranasal surgery—is it necessary? Anaesth Intensive Care 1978;6(4): 328–32.
21. Bromley L, Hayward A. Cocaine absorption from the nasal mucosa. Anaesthesia 1988;43(5):356–8.

# Nuances of Profile Management: The Radix

Jacob D. Steiger, MD*, Shan R. Baker, MD

**KEYWORDS**

• Nuance • Profile • Management • Radix • Rhinoplasty

As rhinoplasty has evolved from its reductive origins, the notion of nasal augmentation has become a fundamental principle within primary and secondary procedures. Modern rhinoplasty surgeons have the skills to perform effective nasal augmentation, which may be combined with or used in lieu of reductive techniques. These surgical skills represent advancement in surgical techniques and have been aided by a philosophic shift in the approach to rhinoplasty. Using these tools, a more balanced and natural-appearing outcome may be achieved.

Profile refinement is one of the most common reasons patients seek consultation for rhinoplasty. Emphasis on creating a natural-appearing nasal dorsum demands a methodic nasal and facial analysis. Areas of dorsal excess and deficiency are identified, quantitated, and considered when determining surgical goals. The radix is an essential component of the profile and is carefully assessed from the standpoint of projection and position. Radix position profoundly impacts the appearance of the nasal profile by influencing dorsal length, contour, angulation, and height. When the radix is ideal in position and projection, rhinoplasty requires that the dorsal line be adjusted in relation to the radix. This adjustment may require modification of the remaining dorsal line using reduction, augmentation, or a combination of these procedures. The goal of this modification is to create a straight profile or one with an appropriate supratip break, depending on the patient's desire. Theoretically, it may be preferable to establish an ideal projection of the nasal tip and radix and then modify the remaining dorsum; however, the senior author finds it more practical to establish an ideal height of the bony and cartilagenous dorsum and then adjust tip and radix projection. To achieve ideal nasal tip projection, augmentation of the alar cartilages may be necessary using struts or grafts, depending on the necessary degree of increased projection. In contrast, to reduce tip projection, the length of the alar cartilages may require shortening when a less invasive procedure is inadequate.

Similar to adjusting tip projection, the surgeon should also adjust the position and projection of the radix when it is not ideal. An overprojected radix is deepened using an osteotome or an electric-powered drill system. In these situations, the bony dorsum is always overprojected, so for practical reasons, the bony dorsum is lowered first or concomitantly with lowering of the radix. A caudally positioned radix is usually associated with an underprojected dorsum. In these circumstances, the entire dorsum is augmented using a bone or cartilage graft sufficient to provide proper height to the nasal bridge and to position the nasofrontal angle cephalically. A deep underprojected radix is corrected with a radix graft. Similar to an overprojected radix, when the bony dorsum requires reduction, it is preferable to reduce the dorsum before grafting the radix. Adjusting the nasal profile to a well-positioned radix leads to a natural and attractive nasal profile.

## ANALYSIS OF THE NASAL PROFILE

The nasal profile consists of the osseocartilagenous dorsum and the nasal tip and their interface with the glabella and subnasale. The profile is defined by its contour, height, length, and interfacing angles. These individual characteristics are not only used to describe the appearance of the profile

Department of Otolaryngology, Center for Facial Cosmetic Surgery, University of Michigan, 19900 Haggerty Road, Suite 103, Livonia, MI 48152, USA
* Corresponding author.
*E-mail address:* jdsteiger@gmail.com (J.D. Steiger).

Facial Plast Surg Clin N Am 17 (2009) 15–28
doi:10.1016/j.fsc.2008.09.007

as a whole but also have a profound impact on each other.

The osseocartilagenous dorsum extends cephalad to the tip-defining point, ending at the nasion. The contour of the dorsal profile should be relatively straight and 1 to 2 mm below a line drawn from the nasion to the tip. This contour imparts the presence of a subtle break in the supratip region. Contour variations may exist based on aesthetic taste, sex, ethnicity, and race. Generally, the ideal male nasal profile may be slightly convex at the rhinion, whereas a slight concavity is desirable in female patients.

The authors use the terms *dorsal height* and *dorsal projection* interchangeably. The terms refer to the overall height of the dorsal nasal profile line from nasion to the tip-defining point. Projection or height of the profile is assessed at the nasion, the rhinion, and the tip-defining point, measured in the Frankfort horizontal plane (**Fig. 1**). The height at the nasion is measured from the anterior corneal plane. Ideal height of the nasion is between 9 mm and 14 mm.[1] The vertical alar plane is used as

a reference for measure of dorsal height/projection at the rhinion and nasal tip. This plane runs tangentially through the alar facial sulcus, perpendicular to the Frankfort horizontal. As measured from this line, ideal dorsal height at the rhinion is between 18 mm and 22 mm, whereas ideal nasal tip projection is between 28 mm and 32 mm.[2] As a rule of thumb, the senior author uses the rule of 10-20-30:[2] 10 mm at the nasion, 20 mm at the rhinion, and 30 mm at the tip.

Important angles to consider when assessing the nasal profile include the nasofacial, nasofrontal, and the nasolabial angles. The nasofacial angle defines nasal projection from the face. It is formed by the intersection of two lines. One line is drawn from the nasion to the pronasalae (tip-defining point) and the other is drawn from the nasion to the pogonion (**Fig. 2**).[3] Ideally, the angle formed by these two lines is 36°. A more acute angle bestows the appearance of increased nasal length, whereas more obtuse angles contribute to the appearance of a shorter, more projected nose. The nasofrontal angle is the obtuse angle between a line tangent to the glabella and a line tangent to the pronasalae, with both lines originating at

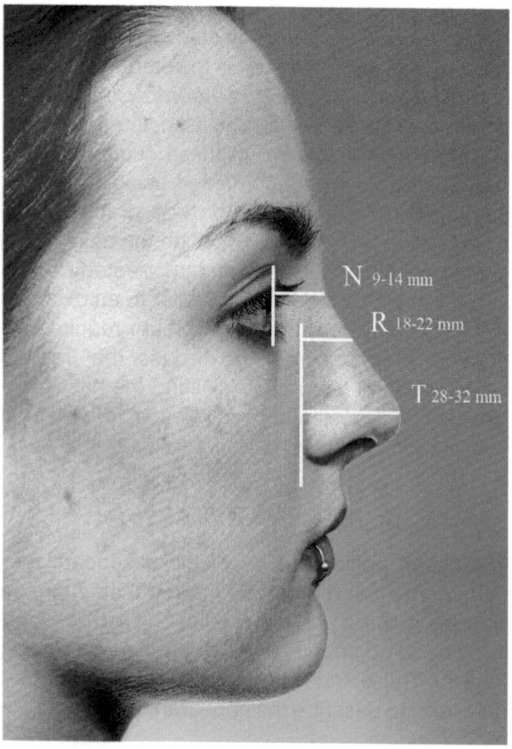

**Fig. 1.** Measuring nasal height. Nasal height is measured at the nasion (N), rhinion (R), and tip-defining point (T) (pronasalae). The reference of origin for the nasion begins at the anterior corneal plane, whereas the vertical alar plane is referenced when measuring rhinion height and tip projection. Standard averages for each region are shown.

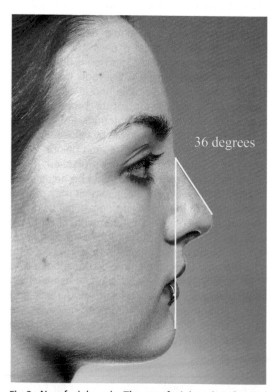

**Fig. 2.** Nasofacial angle. The nasofacial angle is formed by the intersection of two lines. One line is drawn from nasion to pronasalae and the other is drawn from nasion to pogonion. Ideally, this angle approximates 36°.

the nasion. This angle is ideally between 115° and 135° (**Fig. 3**). The nasolabial angle is the angle formed between the plane of the columella and upper lip as seen on profile. Ideally, it measures between 105° and 115° in female patients and between 90° and 105° in male patients.

The cephalocaudal position of the radix directly affects the nasofacial angle. As the radix is positioned cephalad, the nasofacial angle becomes more acute. A caudally positioned radix opens the nasofacial angle and increases relative nasal projection. Thus, the position of the radix has a significant impact on the overall appearance and balance of the nasal profile and must be considered in the surgical plan.

Nasal length is the distance from the nasion to the nasal tip, which ideally is between 45 mm and 49 mm.[1] Numerous methods of estimating the ideal length have been described. Byrd and Hobar[1] suggested that ideal nasal length should equal two thirds of the height of the midface, as measured from the glabella to the subnasale. Other methods of determining length involve ratios that describe the ideal nasal shape. These ratios involve the relation between nasal length, height, tip projection,

and angulation. Crumley and Lancer[3] stated that the ideal nasal profile forms a 3:4:5 right triangle. Goode's method calls for a ratio of 0.55:0.60 between tip projection and nasal length (**Fig. 4**).[4] Both methods mathematically infer a nasofacial angle of approximately 36° degrees. Although there is no substitute for the aesthetic eye, the aforementioned measurements, ratios, and angles serve as guidelines toward surgical planning.

### The Radix

The nasion is a depression at the root of the nose corresponding to the nasofrontal suture. The sellion is the deepest point of the nasofrontal angle at the intersection of forehead slope and the proximal nasal bridge. It is the soft tissue equivalent of the nasion. Centered at the nasion, the radix defines the nasal root and represents where the nose has its origin from the glabella. It extends inferiorly from the nasion to the level of a horizontal line passed through the lateral canthi. The radix

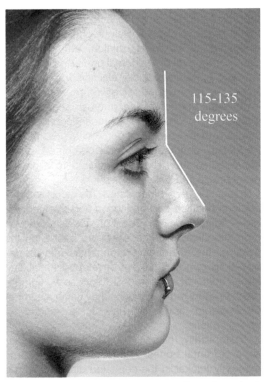

Fig. 3. Nasofrontal angle. The nasofrontal angle is measured at the nasion. It is formed by the intersection at the nasion of lines tangent to the infrabrow glabella and the pronasalae. Ideally, the nasofrontal angle is between 115° and 135°.

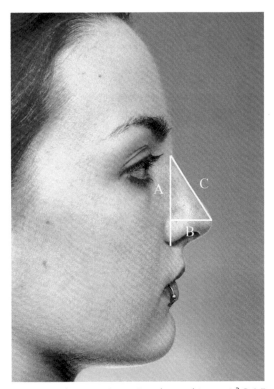

Fig. 4. Nasal proportions. Crumley and Lancer's[3] 3:4:5 right triangle of ideal nasal proportion. This triangle is formed by the vertical tangent between the nasion and alar facial sulcus (A), a perpendicular line from this tangent to the tip-defining point (B), and the dorsal line (C). B:A:C should approximate a 3:4:5 ratio. Goode's method for evaluating appropriate projection relates tip projection to nasal length. The ratio of B:C should approximate 0.55:0.60.

extends superiorly from the nasion for an equivalent distance (**Fig. 5**). The radix is defined by its height and vertical position. At the nasion, the height of the radix is ideally between 9 mm and 14 mm as measured from the anterior corneal plane.[1] When projection of the radix is less than this range, the authors refer to this condition as a low radix. The vertical position of the radix should lie between the level of the supratarsal crease and the superior eyelid lash line.[2] When the vertical position of the radix is inferior to the superior lash line, the authors refer to this as a caudally positioned radix. During rhinoplasty, the surgeon's aesthetic sense ultimately guides the appropriate position of the nasion, taking into consideration the patient's sex, ethnicity, and overall facial appearance, with particular attention to the vertical height of the face. Ideally, the greater the vertical height of the face, the more rostral the position of the radix.

The position of the radix significantly influences the overall balance of the nasal profile. It impacts nasal contour, length, angulation, and height. The radix marks the origin of the nasal dorsum, directly influencing nasal length. Positioning the radix more cephalad has the effect of lengthening the

dorsal line, whereas caudal displacement shortens the nasal length.

Nasal contour is affected by radix position and projection. A "top-heavy nose" is characterized by a rostrally positioned and often overprojected radix with an obtuse nasofrontal angle.[5] This contour is always associated with an overprojected bony vault that causes the casual observer's eyes to be drawn toward the nasal bridge and away from the tip. On the other hand, an underprojected or caudally positioned radix usually diverts the observer's eyes toward the nasal tip, particularly when the nasal base is wide. This combination of a wide nasal base and a narrow underprojected or caudally positioned radix creates imbalance between the cephalic one third and the caudal one third of the nose. A nose with this type of configuration is labeled as "bottom heavy." Depending on its position relative to the dorsum, a low radix may also impart a scooped appearance to the nasal profile or portray the illusion of a pseudohump.

## SURGICAL PLANNING

Planning surgical management of the nasal profile begins by determining the ideal configuration of the nasal bridge using the aforementioned aesthetic nasal principles. Height and contour are evaluated at the radix, rhinion, and nasal tip. Each component of the dorsal profile (nasion, rhinion, and tip) is individually classified as overprojected, underprojected, or of appropriate height. To balance the dorsal line, augmentation and reduction of portions of the osseocartilagenous dorsum are in the realm of corrective possibilities. Reduction, augmentation, or a combined reduction/augmentation may be required to align the nasal profile in a balanced fashion.

In most primary rhinoplasties, the radix is appropriate in position and projection and does not require adjustment. In 20% of cases, however, radix modification is necessary to best align the nasal profile.[2] Reductive techniques may be required to remove the overdeveloped nasal and frontal bones of a high radix. Conversely, augmentation of a low radix is achieved by using a number of available graft materials in a myriad of configurations.

Anatomically, the nasion is composed of the nasal and frontal bones. The nasal bones become markedly thicker in the cephalad direction, as do the overlying nasal skin and soft tissue envelope. The procerus muscle and an increased quantity of subcutaneous fat account for the thickness of the soft tissue in this region. Although helpful for camouflaging imperfect radix grafts, the

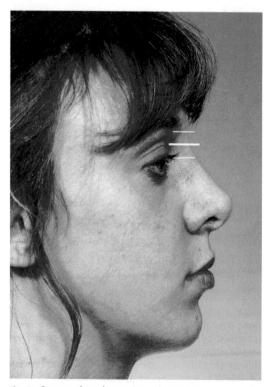

**Fig. 5.** Centered at the nasion, the radix extends inferiorly to the level of the lateral canthus and superiorly by an equivalent distance.

combination of thick skin and soft tissue causes difficulty in precisely assessing reduction or augmentation of the radix. It is also difficult to adequately reduce the projection of the radix because of the dense bone in this area of the nasal bridge. Removal of nasofrontal bone at the radix only translates to approximately 25% of the effective reduction at the surface level (sellion).[6] The surgeon must account for this inefficient translation when planning and executing surgical reduction.

An overprojected radix is often found in the setting of a prominent dorsal hump. Depending on the desired degree of reduction, the radix may be lowered with a rasp, osteotome, or drill bur. When a prominent dorsal hump is present, access to the radix is best achieved by first reducing the osseocartilagenous dorsum. In an open rhinoplasty approach, an Aufricht retractor assists in exposing the radix and allows for reduction under direct visualization. Although minor reductions of the caudal portion of the radix may be achieved with a rasp, substantial reductions necessitate more aggressive techniques. A wedge resection of the nasofrontal bones with an osteotome is often effective in reducing the projection of the radix and in deepening the nasofrontal angle. If the radix is overdeveloped from significant frontal bone contribution, drilling down the bone with a guarded burr is required to produce effective change and is accomplished under direct visualization through an open rhinoplasty approach. When more extensive surgical dissection is performed, appreciable improvement in reduction and angulation of the radix will take several months to reveal itself as edema of the thick skin and soft tissue subsides.

An overprojected or convex dorsum is the most frequently encountered deformity in primary rhinoplasty. Evaluation of the radix in relation to the dorsum reveals the best method for a balanced profile plasty. A deep radix may bestow the appearance of a pseudohump to an otherwise appropriate dorsal height. A deep radix may also accentuate an existing dorsal convexity. In these situations, dorsal reduction instead of or without the addition of radix augmentation results in an overresected nasal bridge and the stigmata of a "surgical" nose. To achieve balanced correction, the radix must first be set to the ideal position and projection. When set, further reduction of the dorsum may or may not be required to align the nasal profile.

Augmentation of the radix may be achieved with grafts assembled from autogenous or alloplastic material. Septal cartilage is frequently used because of its durability, effectiveness, and availability within the surgical field. When septal cartilage is insufficient or unavailable, the surgeon may turn to other autografts such as auricular cartilage, costal cartilage, or native soft tissue. Graft visibility remains the most significant risk of using cartilage to augment the radix. Depending on personal preference and cartilage availability, alloplastic implants are viable alternatives for augmentation of the radix. Although the risks associated with alloplastic nasal implants remain a significant concern, high success rates with minimal complications have been reported with the use of ePTFE (Gore-Tex; W.L. Gore and Associates, Inc., Flagstaff, Arizona) as a radix graft.[7]

The necessary degree of augmentation of the radix directly influences graft selection. Small, 1 mm deficiencies can be corrected with soft tissue grafts inserted within precise pockets beneath the periosteum of the radix. The malleable nature of soft tissue grafts negates the risk of long-term graft visibility, making it an ideal graft in this situation. Greater degrees of augmentation may be achieved with cartilage or bone grafts. Although cartilage is more commonly used than bone, the senior author has often used the resected bony hump for a radix graft. In such cases, the bony convexity consisting of bone and cartilage at the rhinion is resected in one piece using an osteotome. The resected specimen is then moved cephalad into the area of the radix and beneath the periosteum. The composite graft often sits perfectly in the depths of the nasion, having the correct shape and contour for augmenting it.

When using cartilage grafts to augment the radix, grafts are designed as a single layer or are stacked to the appropriate size and shape depending on cartilage thickness and the desired degree of augmentation. The potential for graft visibility is a significant concern, particularly as the graft size increases and in those patients who have thin skin. In the senior author's experience, approximately 5% of cases may require revision surgery to correct graft visibility. Edges are morselized, bruised, or beveled to prevent graft show, especially in patients who have thin skin. The graft is placed within a dissected pocket beneath the periosteum and is reassessed for position, effect, and stability. When the graft is found to be unstable, a transcutaneous suture can secure the graft and prevent postoperative migration. The suture is removed at the first postoperative visit.

Aside from Asian and African American noses, a low dorsum is infrequently encountered in primary rhinoplasty; however, augmentation of a low dorsum is often necessary in revision cases. Depending on the etiology of the deficiency, the radix may also be malpositioned. Augmentation of the radix and dorsum is required in these cases. These deformities may be treated individually with separate grafts but are more commonly corrected simultaneously with a single graft. A single graft has the advantage of providing a smooth, gapless transition between augmented regions, reducing the risk of graft visibility. Single grafts may extend the complete length of the dorsum, extending distally from the radix. An extended radix graft fashioned from a large portion of septal cartilage can augment a deep radix, increasing its projection and cephalic position while augmenting the width and height of the rhinion. The edges of the graft are bruised or tapered to prevent graft visibility, and the graft is placed into a precise pocket beneath the nasal periosteum (**Fig. 6**).

## CASE EXAMPLES
### Case 1

A 27-year-old woman requested reduction of her dorsal convexity (**Fig. 7**). Profile analysis revealed a deep radix, an overprojected rhinion, and normal tip projection. A deep supratip depression created the illusion of an overprojected tip. Surgical

correction included augmentation of the radix and caudal dorsum in the area of the supratip depression and reduction of the rhinion. A double-layered septal cartilage graft was positioned at the radix, and a single piece of septal cartilage was inserted as a small onlay graft in the supratip area of the cartilagenous dorsum. **Fig. 7** shows views at 1.5 years postoperatively. Alignment of the nasal profile in relationship to a properly positioned radix, rhinion, and nasal tip produced a balanced nasal profile. Tip projection was not altered; however, augmentation of the caudal dorsum lessened the supratip break, which had the effect of reducing the apparent tip rotation and creating the appearance of less tip projection. This case illustrates the visual phenomenon of accentuated height of the rhinion caused by a deep radix and an excessive supratip depression.

### Case 2

A 34-year-old woman presented for primary rhinoplasty with concerns centered on the appearance of her nasal profile (**Fig. 8**). Nasal analysis revealed

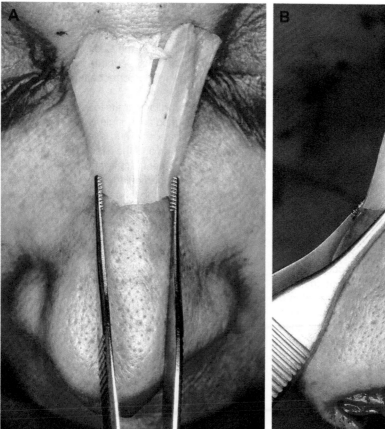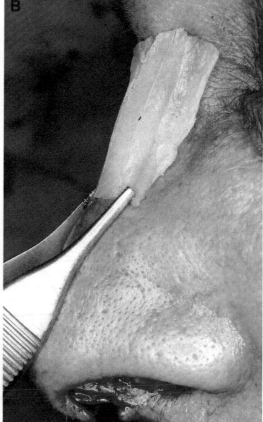

**Fig. 6.** (*A, B*) Extended radix graft fashioned from a large portion of septal cartilage used to augment a narrow underprojected radix and a cephalic bony nasal dorsum. (*C, D*) Profile before and following insertion of extended radix graft.

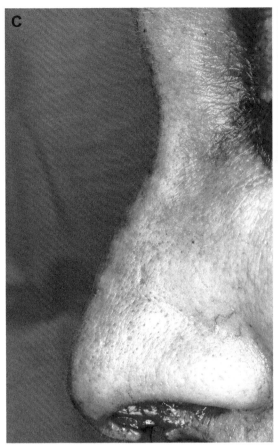

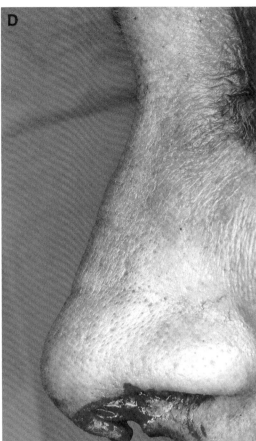

**Fig. 6.** *(continued)*.

a caudally positioned radix, an underprojected osseocartilagenous vault, and normal tip projection. The position of the radix accentuated a slight convexity at the rhinion. The patient also had microgenia. Surgical correction included augmentation of the radix and osseocartilagenous vault with a single-layer septal cartilage graft. The convexity of the rhinion was eliminated to provide a flat surface for placement of the dorsal augmentation graft. A chin implant was inserted for enhancement. Although the tip was rotated cephalad, projection remained unchanged. Dorsal augmentation accounted for the increase in the height of the nasal profile observed 1.5 years postoperatively.

## Case 3

A 58-year-old woman presented for primary rhinoplasty, requesting a smaller nose. Nasal analysis revealed a caudally positioned and underprojected radix, an overprojected rhinion, and an overprojected tip (**Fig. 9**). The entire bony nasal vault was underdeveloped and overly narrow. The nasal tip was greatly overprojected, and the nasal base was excessively wide, creating a typical

"bottom-heavy nose." The patient also exhibited loose redundant nasal skin. The excess nasal skin prevented aggressive reduction of nasal tip projection. Because of these findings, it was elected to augment the width and height of the bony nasal vault and to perform a conservative retro displacement of the tip. The width of the nasal base was also reduced. The bony nasal vault was augmented in width and dorsal height by using a single large septal cartilage graft (see **Fig. 6**). At 1.5 years postoperatively, views reveal a lengthened and more ideal nasal profile (see **Fig. 9**). Without the use of the large radix and bony dorsal graft, greater reduction of the cartilagenous dorsum would have been necessary. Consequently, the nasal tip would have required a comparatively greater degree of retro displacement, which in turn would have resulted in an unnatural and unbalanced nasal profile.

## Case 4

A 35-year-old woman presented for revision rhinoplasty requesting reduction of her "large" nose. Analysis of the nasal profile revealed an

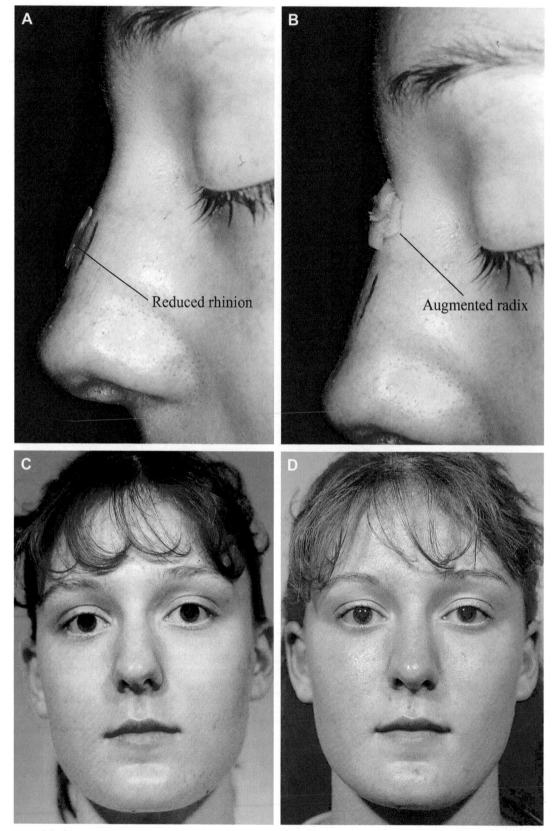

**Fig. 7.** (*A*) Rhinion reduced by 1.5 mm. (*B*) Nasion augmented with septal cartilage graft. (*C–H*) Preoperative and 1.5 years postoperative views.

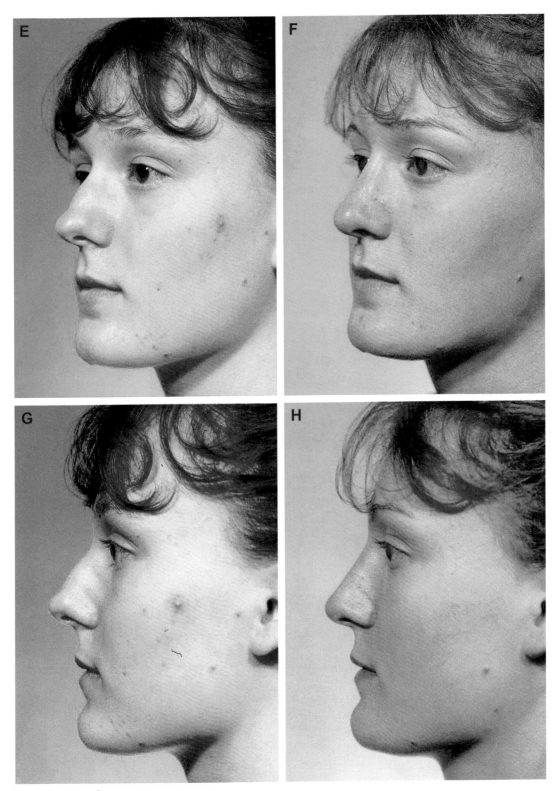

**Fig. 7.** (*continued*).

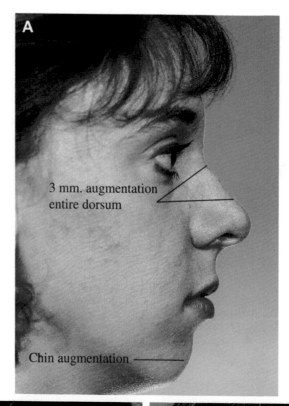

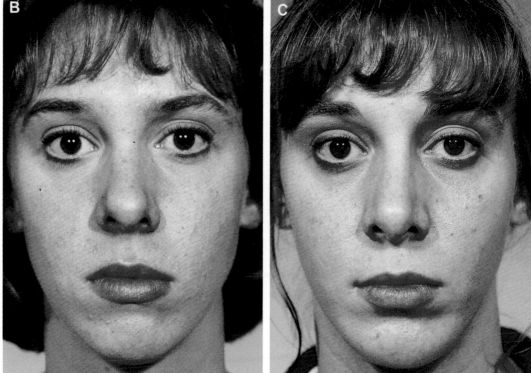

Fig. 8. (A) Entire osseocartilagenous vault is underprojected; radix is underprojected and caudally positioned. Profile plasty was performed using a single dorsal septal cartilage graft. (B–G) Preoperative and 1.5 years postoperative views.

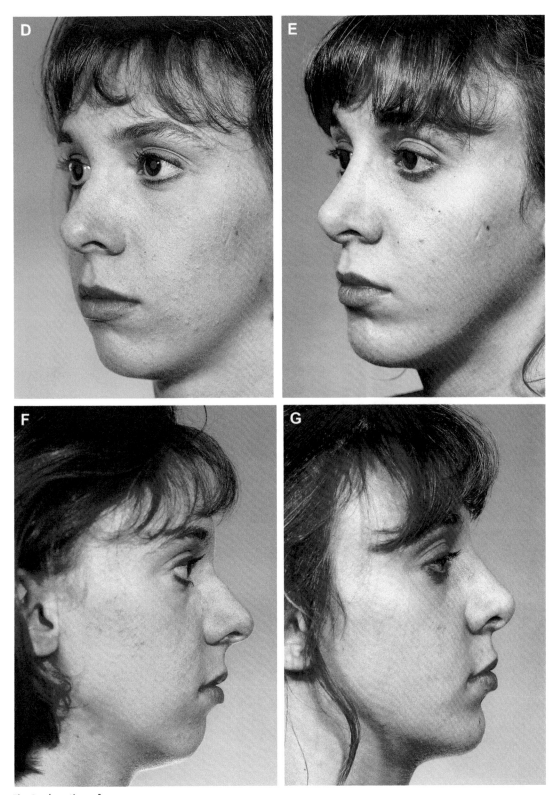

**Fig. 8.** (*continued*).

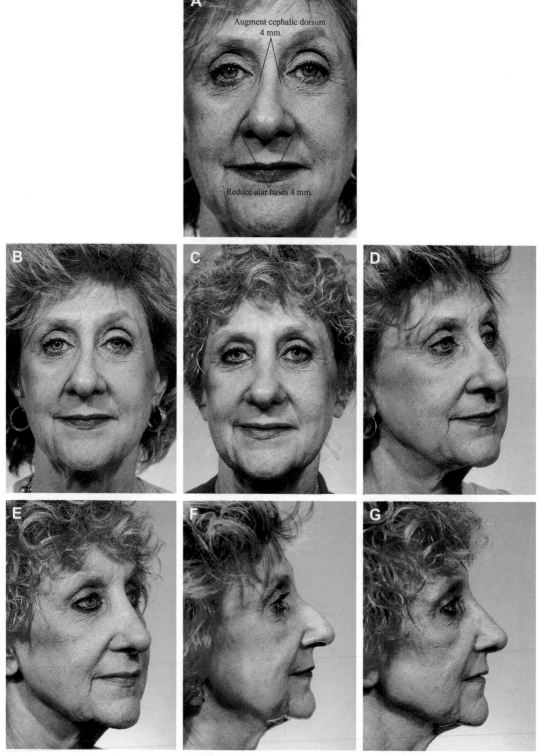

**Fig. 9.** Necessary surgical steps to create a more balanced profile. (*A*) The combination of a wide nasal base and a narrow underprojected radix creates a "bottom-heavy nose." The bony nasal vault was augmented in width and dorsal height using a single large septal cartilage graft. Nasal base was narrowed 8 mm. Projection of nasal tip and caudal nasal dorsum was reduced. (*B–G*) Preoperative and 1.5 years postoperative views.

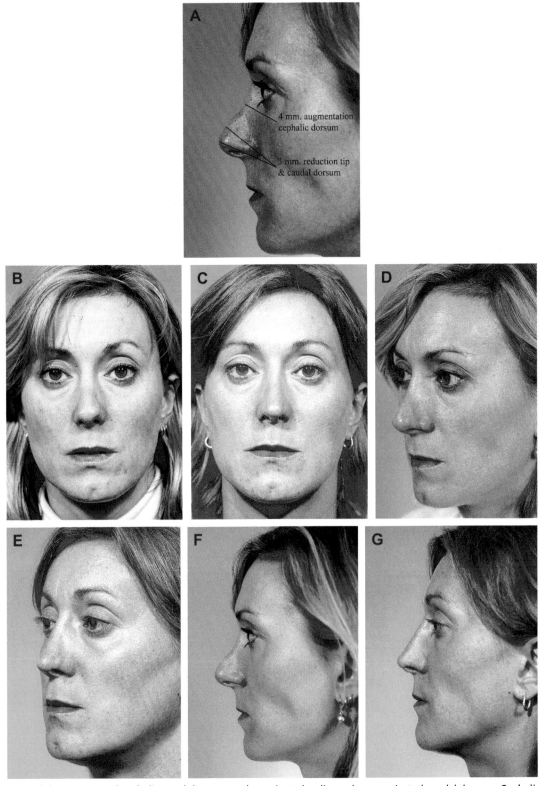

**Fig. 10.** (*A*) Overresected cephalic nasal dorsum, underprojected radix, and overprojected caudal dorsum. Cephalic dorsum and radix were augmented using an alloplastic extended radix implant. (*B–G*) Preoperative and 2 years postoperative views.

inadequate height of the bony dorsum including the radix. This inadequacy was accentuated by excessive projection of the cartilagenous dorsum and nasal tip. The surgeon performing the original rhinoplasty had overresected the cephalic portion of the dorsum while failing to address the overprojected nasal tip and caudal dorsum. Augmentation of the radix and cephalic dorsum was achieved with an alloplastic (Gore-Tex; W.L. Gore and Associates, Inc.) extended radix implant. The caudal dorsum was then aligned to the level of the implant, and the tip was retro displaced. Two-year postoperative views demonstrate a more ideal nasal profile (**Fig. 10**). The radix and dorsal implant reduced the nasofacial angle, lengthened the nose, and restored dorsal height.

## REFERENCES

1. Byrd S, Hobar C. Dimensional rhinoplasty. Plast Reconstr Surg.
2. Rollin KD. Rhinoplasty. 1993.
3. Crumley RL, Lancer R. Quantitative analysis of nasal tip projection. Laryngoscope 1988;98:202–8.
4. Powell N, Humphreys B. Proportions of the aesthetic face. New York: Thieme-Stratton; 1984.
5. Sheen JH, Sheen AP. Aesthetic rhinoplasty. 2nd Edition. St Louis (MO): Mosby; 1987.
6. Guyron B. Precision rhinoplasty. Part II: prediction. Plast Reconstr Surg 1988;81:500.
7. Johnson CM Jr, Alsarraf R. The radix graft in cosmetic rhinoplasty. Arch Facial Plast Surg 2001; 3(2):120–1.

# Nasal Tip Dynamics

Peter A. Adamson, MD, FRCSC, FACS[a],*, Etai Funk, MD[b,c]

## KEYWORDS

- Rhinoplasty • Tripod concept • M-arch model

Rhinoplasty has been described as one of the most challenging procedures in plastic surgery. Gustave Aufricht once said, "Rhinoplasty is an easy operation, it is just difficult to get good results." Although we are well familiar with the plethora of techniques available for manipulation of the nasal tip, the challenge is in knowing when to apply these techniques to achieve the appropriate correction. An intimate knowledge of nasal tip dynamics as they apply to the cartilaginous tip superstructure is most advantageous. One model that has remained steadfast is the tripod concept proposed by Jack R. Anderson in 1969.[1] As is widely known, this concept characterizes the lower lateral cartilages as a tripod whose legs are represented by the two lateral crura and conjoined medial crura. At the time, rhinoplasty was largely a reductive operation and this idea was originally conceived to theoretically describe the effects of tip reduction and rotation maneuvers by shortening of the tripod's legs.

Our levels of knowledge and sophistication with respect to tip refinement have significantly evolved with the popularization of the open rhinoplasty approach[2] and increasing reliance on suture refinement and other preservationist philosophies. Our understanding of tip anatomy has become more nuanced, such as by the introduction and further characterization of the intermediate crura (Fig. 1). It is fitting that, in this more progressive era of rhinoplasty, our concept of tip dynamics must also keep pace to optimally aid in surgical planning and execution.

## NASAL TIP DYNAMICS

There are numerous support structures for the nasal tip that are cartilaginous, ligamentous, and soft tissue–based. The major supporting areas for the tip include the feet of the medial crura where they hug the posterior septal angle, the feet or hinge areas of the lower lateral crura where they are supported by the pyriform margin, the scroll region, and the interdomal ligaments.

The curvature in the conjoined medial and lateral crura, which include the intermediate crura, creates a tension in the structure, somewhat like a sprung horseshoe. The anterior tension in the lower lateral crura makes them project the nasal tip, thrusting it anteriorly and inferiorly. The medial crura counteract this with an anterior and superior thrusting motion (Fig. 2). Soft tissue and ligaments contribute to the balance achieved between these opposing forces, thus determining the tip-defining point in space and the nasal parameters of length, projection, and rotation.

## THE TRIPOD CONCEPT AND THE M-ARCH MODEL

The tripod concept as described by Anderson[1] envisions the conjoined medial crura to form one leg of a tripod and each of the lower lateral crura to form the other two legs. By shortening the medial or lateral crural lengths, the surgeon can alter the position of the tip-defining point. Shortening the legs obviously decreases projection, and depending on the integrated degree of shortening of the medial and lateral crura, there is a variable effect on rotation. The purpose of the tripod concept is to allow one to conceptualize maneuvers that alter tip projection, rotation, and ultimately nasal length.

The tripod concept did not originally consider the effects of lengthening the medial and lateral crural legs. Also, it did not address issues related to its effects on the lobule, columella, alar margin, or base. Nor did it consider the intermediate crus, a term

a Division of Facial Plastic and Reconstructive Surgery, Department of Otolaryngology–Head and Neck Surgery, University of Toronto, Toronto, Ontario, Canada
b The Bressler Center for Facial Plastic Surgery and Skin Care, Houston, TX, USA
c Bobby R. Alford Department of Otolaryngology–Head and Neck Surgery, Baylor College of Medicine, Houston, TX, USA
* Corresponding author.
E-mail address: paa@dradamson.com (P.A. Adamson).

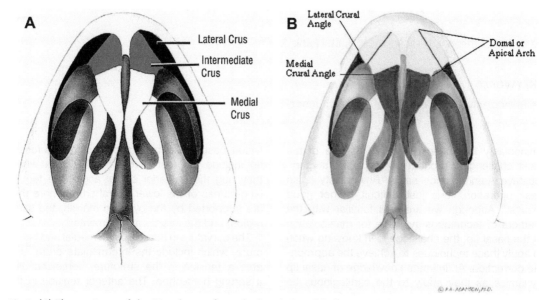

**Fig. 1.** (*A*) The anatomy of the M-arch seen from the basal view. (*B*) The paired domal or apical arches as demonstrated by the yellow portions of the crura. The lobular arch is composed of the paired domal or apical arches.

defined subsequent to the original description of the tripod concept. This concept has stood the test of time mostly because of its simplicity and validity.

The M-arch model has been devised as a modern and more sophisticated extension of the tripod concept with broader applications relative to the major nasal parameters of length, projection, and rotation. It also integrates maneuvers that are applicable to create ideal lobule definition.[3,4] The M-arch model considers the entire tip tripod as an arch that is shaped like the letter "M." The components of this anatomic arch are the paired medial, intermediate, and lateral crura. Furthermore, the M-arch model defines the lobular arch, which is an arch within the M-arch. This lobular arch is constituted anatomically by the paired, bilateral intermediate crura and anterior-most aspect of the

lateral crura. The lobular arch is defined aesthetically as the infratip, supratip, and lateral tip lobule. It is the refinement of this lobular arch that creates the ideal lobule aesthetic in rhinoplasty.

Another anatomic arch within the M-arch is the domal or apical arch, of which there are two, one on each side. The domal arch is formed unilaterally by the intermediate crus and anterior aspect of the lateral crus. The conjoined domal arches constitute the lobular arch.

Another defining distinction of the M-arch model is the concept that the M-arch cannot only be shortened, as in the tripod concept, but can also be lengthened. Either shortening or lengthening alters nasal length, tip projection, and rotation.

Although the tripod concept predicts a uniform effect on tip rotation and projection for a given shortening maneuver, the M-arch model, by contrast, recognizes that an equal amount of shortening or lengthening of the M-arch may produce variable yet predictable changes in these nasal parameters, depending on where the arch is shortened. For example, shortening of the medial crura causes deprojection and counter-rotation, whereas shortening of the lateral crus causes deprojection and rotation. Shortening the intermediate crus causes a variable degree of deprojection and rotation depending on where the vertical division and overlap is performed. If done near the angle, at the junction of the medial and intermediate crus, there is more deprojection and less rotation. If done closer to the apex of the apical arch, there is more rotation and less deprojection (**Fig. 3**).

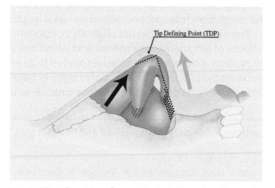

**Fig. 2.** The thrusting forces that define the dynamics of the M-arch. Thrusting forces are depicted by arrows. The tip-defining point is determined by the resultant thrusting forces and the intrinsic lobule shape.

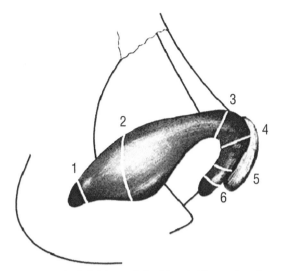

Fig. 3. Vertical divisions of the M-arch. The various locations that have been described as sites to divide the M-arch: (1) hinge area, (2) lateral crural flap, (3) Goldman maneuver, (4) vertical lobule division, (5) Lipsett maneuver, and (6) medial crural feet.

In lengthening the medial, intermediate, or lateral crura with cartilage advancements or grafts, projection can be increased and rotation can be increased or decreased depending on the location of graft placement. For example, an infratip shield graft provides projection and counter-rotation, whereas a cap graft creates projection and apparent rotation of the lobule.

The M-arch model further recognizes that these changes can effect lobular refinement, something not addressed with the initial tripod concept. For example, shortening of the intermediate crura shortens the length of the infratip lobule and increases the angle of the domal arch, thereby rounding the external soft tissue triangle. If the vertical division of the intermediate crus is performed near the angle or junction of the medial crura and intermediate crura, a hanging infratip lobule can be reduced. If done near the apex of the domal arch, a boxy or biconvex lobular arch can be narrowed.

## APPLICATIONS OF THE M-ARCH MODEL

In assessing the nasal tip, the first analysis is to determine the lengths of the medial, intermediate, and lateral crura. In many instances, the length of the M-arch may be deemed satisfactory—that is, not too long or too short relative to the ideal nasal length, projection, and rotation that is being sought. If only lobular refinement is necessary, and can be achieved through conservative horizontal cephalic lateral crura resection and suturing techniques, then nothing more need be done. But if it is deemed

that lobular refinement, or the length, projection, or rotation of the nose, requires changing the M-arch in any of its three anatomic components (medial, intermediate, or lateral crura), then the appropriate place where the M-arch is to be changed in length must be determined.

### Shortening a Long M-arch

A minor degree of deprojection can be achieved by weakening of nasal tip supports, such as by a full transfixion incision or by shortening of the caudal septum or nasal spine. These techniques may destabilize the nasal tip and lead to a pollybeak deformity postoperatively if the medial crura are not restabilized with a columellar strut. In addition, they may lack the efficacy to achieve the desired degree of deprojection when the M-arch is excessively long. By shortening the excessive cartilage length of the M-arch directly, there is greater potential for achieving adequate deprojection, more predictable healing outcomes, and preservation or even strengthening of the tip complex.

Vertical division of the M-arch with overlapping suture stabilization of the divided segments provides the most desirable and effective outcome.[5] The location for arch division depends on the desired result. If lobular definition is satisfactory and the goal is to deproject, division at the lateral or medial crural feet preserves lobular contour and rotates or counter-rotates, respectively. For even greater rotational effects, the lateral crural flap (lateral crural overlay) may be performed;[6] this also deprojects the nose. The authors prefer this location for division in most cases, rather than the hinge area, because it minimizes the risk for lateral crural inflaring into the nasal vestibule and potential nasal airway obstruction.

Alternatively, when the lobular contour is asymmetric, vertical division within the domal arch segment may be used to simultaneously correct arch length and asymmetry in addition to irregularities of the lobular-columellar relationship, such as a hanging infratip. Vertical arch divisions are ideally performed within the intermediate crus so that the overlap is concealed in the infratip region postoperatively. This overlap also acts to strengthen any weakened, knuckled, or buckled cartilage (**Fig. 4**). Division nearest the angle of the medial and intermediate crura produces deprojection and vertical M-arch shortening without substantively affecting lobular width or rotation (**Fig. 5A**). Conversely, division nearest the tip-defining point primarily achieves M-arch shortening with narrowing of the lobule (**Fig. 5B**).

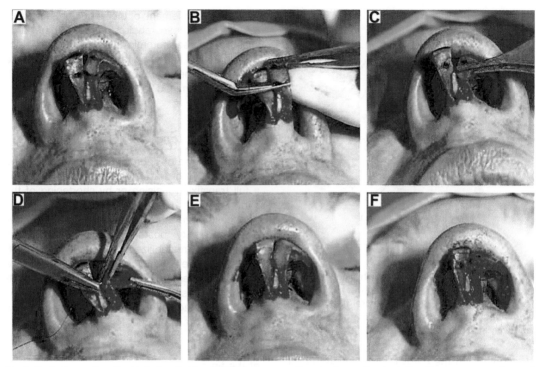

**Fig. 4.** Technique of vertical lobular division (VLD). Intraoperative photographs depicting the sequence of steps in VLD. (*A*) Site of the VLD shown marked. (*B*) Scissors shown cutting through the intermediate crus. (*C*) Overlapped cartilage ends. (*D*) Overlapped ends being sutured. (*E*) Pre-VLD basal view. (*F*) Post-VLD basal view showing a shortened M-arch on the left with resultant deprojection.

These maneuvers may be complemented with tip suturing techniques, such as single dome unit sutures to individually narrow each domal arch and double dome unit or interdomal sutures to medialize the domal arches and thereby narrow the lobular arch (**Fig. 6**).[7,8] Gentle scoring may help with tip definition but should be done cautiously to avoid too much weakening. Horizontal cephalic resection may achieve a small measure of lobule definition and rotation but should also be performed conservatively to avoid postoperative and long-term alar retraction and collapse.

### Lengthening the M-arch

Similarly, the M-arch may be used to predict gains in tip projection. Increasing the medial-intermediate crural segment at the expense of the lateral crural segment to increase projection was traditionally accomplished using the Goldman technique with vertical division lateral to the tip-defining point. This maneuver can sometimes lead to long-term bossa formation, an irregular appearance, and tip instability with healing. It is not the authors' preferred technique, but is performed by some surgeons with good results. Suture and grafting maneuvers are used more often today by the

authors to increase tip projection. The lateral crural steal suturing technique increases the length of the intermediate crura by "borrowing" from the lower lateral crus.[9] Lobular grafts achieve improvements in projection by adding apparent length or vertical height to the M-arch. These can take various forms, depending on the size and shape required to achieve an ideal lobule aesthetic. Some of the common grafts used include the shield or infratip graft, cap graft, buttress graft, interdomal spacer graft, domal underlay, alar strut graft, alar batten graft, and alar margin graft.

The infratip lobule or shield graft is usually placed to provide increased projection and lobule definition, but can also provide counter-rotation and increased nasal length (**Fig. 7**).[10]

The cap (cartilage augmentation-projection) graft, as either a single graft spanning the entire lobule or unilaterally placed on the domal arch, increases projection and possibly definition, depending on its size and shape (**Fig. 8**).

The buttress graft can be placed behind the infratip lobule graft to create more counter-rotation, better lobule definition, and increased nasal length.

The interdomal spacer graft, placed between the intermediate crura, can be used to widen the dome if the tip-defining points are too narrow.[11]

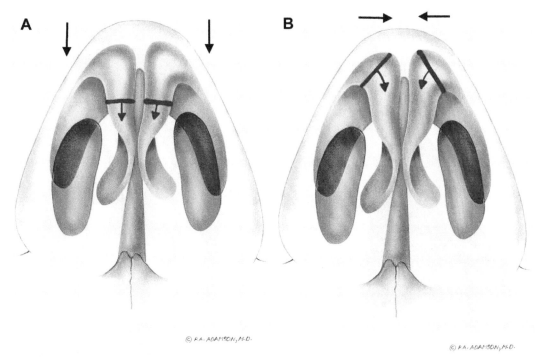

© R.A. ADAMSON, M.D.

© R.A. ADAMSON, M.D.

**Fig. 5.** How vertical lobular division can alter the lobule. (*A*) Here the division and overlap is performed where there is a significant vertical component to the arch, effecting deprojection of the lobule. (*B*) Note that the division and overlap is performed in the arch where there is a significant horizontal component to the arch, effecting a narrowing of the lobule.

A domal underlay graft is similar to an alar strut graft, in that it is laid on the vestibular rather than the dorsal aspect of the apical arch. This graft can be used to create a more natural curve to the dome and strengthen it, especially in cases of knuckling.

The alar strut graft is placed on the vestibular, or underside, of the lower lateral crus to strengthen it.[12] It can be effective in decreasing functional collapse when placed over the pyriform fossa and in improving contour irregularities of the lower lateral crus.

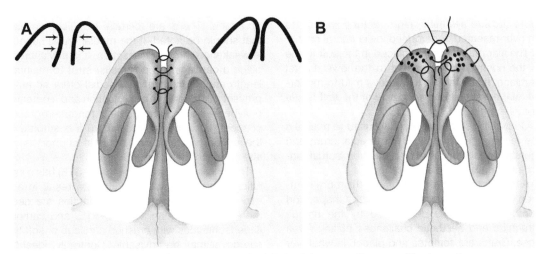

**Fig. 6.** Placement of sutures to define and narrow the lobule. (*A*) Intermediate crural horizontal mattress sutures. (*B*) Single dome unit and interdomal sutures.

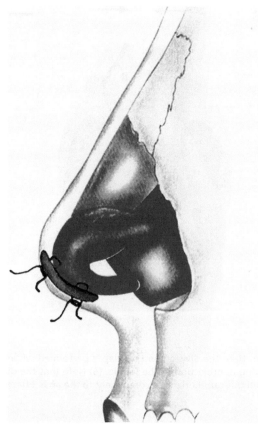

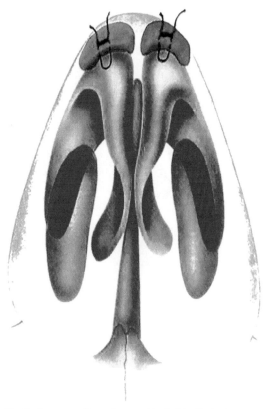

**Fig. 7.** An infratip lobule (shield) graft can be used to increase projection of the nasal tip. As shown, it also creates a slight degree of counter-rotation and increased length.

**Fig. 8.** A cap graft can be used individually to increase projection as a single graft for both domes or separate grafts for each dome.

The alar batten graft is placed on the lateral aspect of the lower lateral crus and is especially useful to provide aesthetic and structural support to an over-resected or deformed lower lateral crus.[13]

The alar margin graft is placed in the soft tissue at the nostril margin, caudal to the lower lateral cartilage. It is effective to improve mild to moderate alar retraction and concavity of the soft tissue nostril margin.[14]

Columellar struts are routinely used to maintain the length and strength of the medial crura and thereby uphold the nasal tip projection, actually increasing arch length and strength.

Although the above are some of the more commonly used nasal tip grafts, the size, shape, and number of grafts is determined by the unique structural and aesthetic challenges of any given nose. Grafts are sculpted and placed in whatever fashion required to achieve maximal improvement, both structurally and aesthetically.

## CAVEATS

Virtually all of these techniques can be applied using either the open or endonasal approach. The more complex the tip deformity and the more complex the surgical techniques applied, the more benefit may be obtained by using an open approach. There are certain technical caveats that should be noted. If the medial crural support is weakened through dissection, it is advisable to place a cartilaginous columellar strut to maintain length and strength of the medial crura so as to prevent postoperative deprojection and a potential pollybeak deformity. The tongue-in-groove concept, in which the medial crura is sutured to the caudal septum for additional support is an alternative to the columellar strut.[15]

The skin–soft tissue envelope (S-STE) has a significant role to play in the ultimate result in any rhinoplasty. Any cartilage irregularities are seen more readily through a thin S-STE, and camouflage techniques with crushed cartilage or soft tissue cover may be advisable. Contrarily, ideal tip definition may be difficult to achieve in a thick-skinned nose wherein conservative thinning of

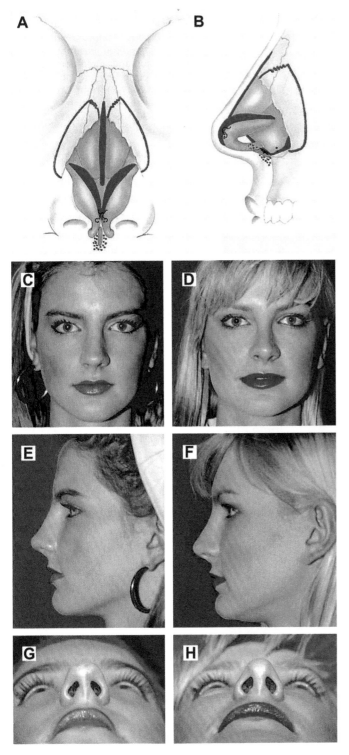

**Fig. 9.** Procedural illustrations (*A, B*) and presurgical (*C, E, G*) and postsurgical (*D, F, H*) patient photographs. Operative schematics (*A, B*) illustrating interdomal suture for refinement of lobule bifidity. Arch length did not require correction. Frontal (*C, D*), left lateral (*E, F*), and basal (*G, H*) views before and 1 year after rhinoplasty.

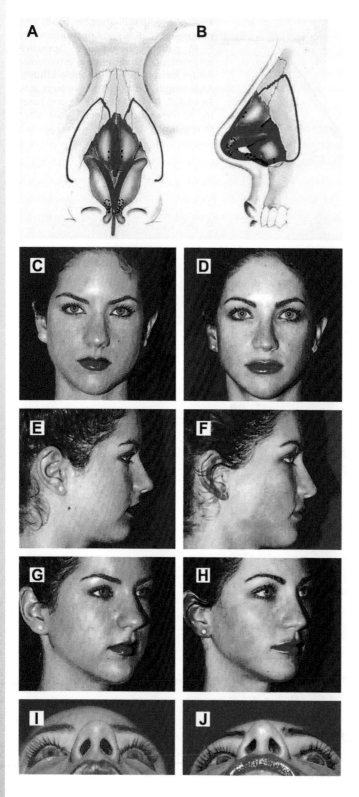

**Fig. 10.** Procedural illustrations (A, B) and presurgical (C, E, G, I) and postsurgical (D, F, H, J) patient photographs. Operative schematics (A, B) illustrating vertical lobule division and single dome unit sutures for deprojection and lobule refinement. Frontal (C, D), right lateral (E, F), right oblique (G, H), and basal (I, J) views before and 30 months after rhinoplasty.

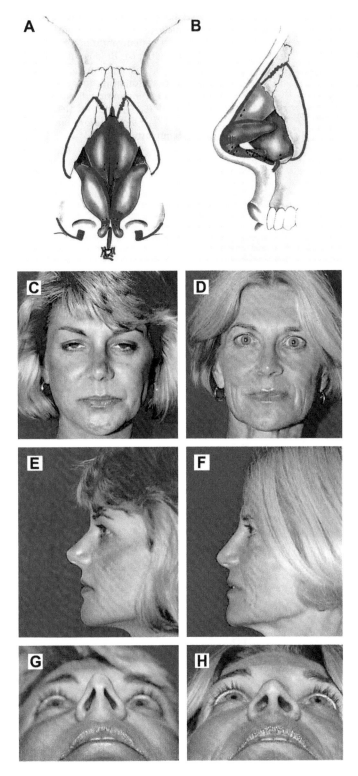

Fig. 11. Procedural illustrations (*A, B*) and presurgical (*C, E, G*) and postsurgical (*D, F, H*) patient photographs. Operative schematics (*A, B*) illustrating vertical lobule division and hinge setback for deprojection and correction of retrusé tip. Frontal (*C, D*), left lateral (*E, F*), and basal (*G, H*) views before and 16 years after rhinoplasty.

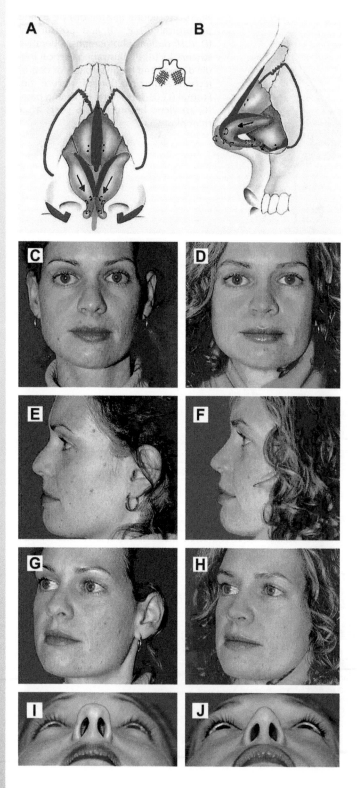

Fig. 12. Procedural illustrations (*A*, *B*) and presurgical (*C*, *E*, *G*, *I*) and postsurgical (*D*, *F*, *H*, *J*) patient photographs. Operative schematics (*A*, *B*) illustrating lateral crural steal, infratip lobule, and buttress/cap graft for projection, counter-rotation, and tip definition. Frontal (*C*, *D*), left lateral (*E*, *F*), left oblique (*G*, *H*), and basal (*I*, *J*) views before and 1 year after rhinoplasty.

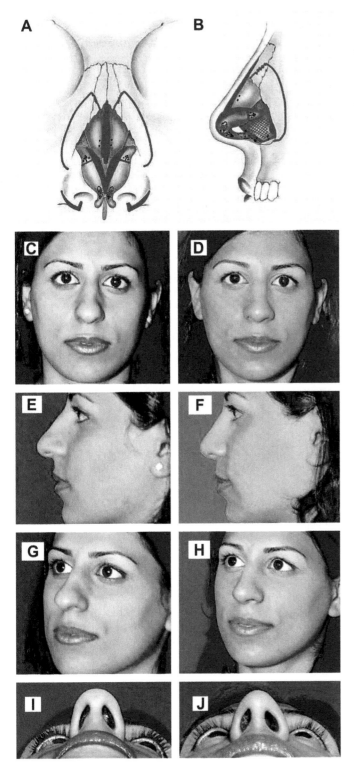

Fig. 13. Procedural illustrations (*A*, *B*) and presurgical (*C*, *E*, *G*, *I*) and postsurgical (*D*, *F*, *H*, *J*) patient photographs. Operative schematics (*A*, *B*) illustrating lateral crural flap, vertical lobule division, and single dome unit sutures for rotation, deprojection, and lobule refinement. Frontal (*C*, *D*), left lateral (*E*, *F*), left oblique (*G*, *H*), and basal (*I*, *J*) views before and 1 year after rhinoplasty. (*From* Adamson PA, Litner JA. Applications of the M-arch model in nasal tip refinement. Facial Plast Surg 2006;22:45; with permission.)

the subcutaneous soft tissue or scar, but never the dermis or subdermal plexus of vessels, may improve definition. This technique becomes somewhat of a double-edged sword because the thicker the S-STE, the greater the cartilage strength must be to support this envelope, and seemingly paradoxically, more cartilage grafting of the lobule may be required to achieve ideal definition.

## SUMMARY

For many years, the tripod concept has been used successfully by rhinoplasty surgeons to conceptualize desired alterations in the positioning of the tip-defining point. Rhinoplasty has evolved in recent decades, however, such that today there are a myriad of techniques available to the rhinoplasty surgeon for tip modification. Just as these techniques have evolved, our theory about nasal tip dynamics must follow. The M-arch model is an extension of, and departure from, the tripod concept. It takes into consideration the overall length of the tip arch, including the intermediate crura. Changes in the length of the arch can be effected at any point within it through suture techniques, grafting, and vertical arch divisions. These techniques can be powerful maneuvers when applied in a graduated and integrated fashion to achieve an ideal aesthetic result (**Figs. 9–13**). The M-arch model provides an efficient evaluative tool for assessment and planning of these maneuvers to effect changes in tip projection, rotation, nasal length, and lobule refinement. We have found the M-arch model to be exceptionally valuable in rhinoplasty planning and in achieving desired aesthetic results.

## REFERENCES

1. Goodman WS, Charbonneau PA. External approach to rhinoplasty. Laryngoscope 1974;84:2195–201.
2. Goodman WS. External approach to rhinoplasty. Can J Otolaryngol 1973;2:207–10.
3. Adamson PA, Litner JA. Applications of the M-arch model in nasal tip refinement. Facial Plast Surg 2006;22:42–8.
4. Adamson PA, Litner JA, Dahiya R. The M-arch model: a new concept of nasal tip dynamics. Arch Facial Plast Surg 2006;8:16–25.
5. Adamson PA, McGraw-Wall BL, Morrow TA, et al. Vertical dome division in open rhinoplasty. An update on indications, techniques, and results. Arch Otolaryngol Head Neck Surg 1994;120: 373–80.
6. Foda HM, Kridel RW. Lateral crural steal and lateral crural overlay: an objective evaluation. Arch Otolaryngol Head Neck Surg 1999;125: 1365–70.
7. Behmand RA, Ghavami A, Guyuron B. Nasal tip sutures part I: the evolution. Plast Reconstr Surg 2003;112:1125–9 [discussion: 46–9].
8. Guyuron B, Behmand RA. Nasal tip sutures part II: the interplays. Plast Reconstr Surg 2003;112: 1130–45 [discussion: 46–9].
9. Kridel RW, Konior RJ, Shumrick KA, et al. Advances in nasal tip surgery. The lateral crural steal. Arch Otolaryngol Head Neck Surg 1989; 115:1206–12.
10. Kamer FM, Churukian MM. Shield graft for the nasal tip. Arch Otolaryngol 1984;110:608–10.
11. Rheims DM, Meyer R. [Alar and columellar refinement in rhinoplasty]. Ann Chir Plast Esthet 1989; 34:141–5.
12. Gunter JP, Friedman RM. Lateral crural strut graft: technique and clinical applications in rhinoplasty. Plast Reconstr Surg 1997;99:943–52 [discussion: 53–5].
13. Otley CC. Alar batten cartilage grafting. Dermatol Surg 2000;26:969–72.
14. Toriumi DM. New concepts in nasal tip contouring. Arch Facial Plast Surg 2006;8:156–85.
15. Kridel RW, Scott BA, Foda HM. The tongue-in-groove technique in septorhinoplasty. A 10-year experience. Arch Facial Plast Surg 1999;1:246–56 [discussion: 57–8].

# Endonasal Suture Techniques in Tip Rhinoplasty

Stephen Perkins, MD[a,b], Amit Patel, MD[b],*

**KEYWORDS**

- Endonasal suture • Tip rhinoplasty
- Favorable tip contour • Double-dome concept
- Individual deformities

Surgical improvement of the broad nasal tip presents a formidable challenge to the rhinoplasty surgeon.[1] The variety of deformities that fall under this category (ie, boxy, bifid, bulbous, trapezoid, amorphous) are generally characterized by excessive width of the alar cartilage complex. In many cases, this excess width is the result of an inherent convexity of the lower lateral cartilages, an overly obtuse domal or interdomal angle, cephalic positioning of the lower lateral cartilages, or a combination of these characteristics.[2,3] The ultimate goal for surgical correction of this type of deformity is to narrow the tip contour without compromising nasal function (ie, airway compromise secondary to internal recurvature of the lower lateral cartilage) (**Box 1**).

Nasal tip–shaping approaches and techniques have evolved significantly in the last few decades.[1] Earlier philosophies favored an excision-based style that supported aggressive scoring and resection of alar cartilages. Unfortunately, excessive resection frequently resulted in a loss of nasal tip support, with the subsequent risk for contour deformities and functional compromise. Such observation has underlined the importance of respecting the major and minor tip support mechanisms in surgical planning.[4]

The era of open structure rhinoplasty that subsequently followed has focused more on cartilage preservation and has emphasized the use of various grafts for contouring. Grafting techniques used to improve lobular definition have come to play an important role in more advanced nasal surgery. These techniques, however, also carry an inherent set of risks by introducing an additional variable to the healing process, and thus the ultimate aesthetic outcome. Graft visibility or migration, particularly in thin-skinned patients, is a potential complication that increases the risk for secondary deformity.

Cartilage suturing techniques, on the other hand, provide a reliable alternative for tip modification. Various sutures can be used to reshape the alar cartilage complex by

> Narrowing inherent convexities to reduce tip width
> Repositioning its spatial relationship to the caudal septum, thereby modifying rotation and projection
> Controlling which areas project into the skin–soft tissue envelope for balancing tip highlights and shadows

Such modifications are made using the existing tip anatomy while still preserving the key structural support mechanisms.

The senior author has found the single- and double-dome suture techniques to be extremely versatile for correction of the broad nasal tip.[5] The soft, pliable character of the native alar cartilages reduces the need for camouflaging maneuvers that may otherwise be required when cartilage contour grafts are used exclusively. The reversible nature of the double-dome technique further

a Department of Otolaryngology–Head and Neck Surgery, Indiana University School of Medicine, Indianapolis, IN, USA
b Meridian Plastic Surgeons and Medical Skin Care, 170 West 106th Street, Indianapolis, IN, USA
* Corresponding author.
E-mail address: apatelfps@gmail.com (A. Patel).

Facial Plast Surg Clin N Am 17 (2009) 41–54
doi:10.1016/j.fsc.2008.10.004

---

**Box 1**
**Operative effects achieved with sutured double-dome tip surgery**

Define and narrow the bulbous, broad, or amorphous tip

Correct and narrow the boxy tip

Efface bifidity

Approximate divergent intermediate crura

Provide strength to soft lobular cartilages

Increase tip support

Increase tip projection

Correct asymmetries and length of crural disparity

---

allows precise control during tip sculpting. By varying the suture orientation, the surgeon can predictably guide tip projection, rotation, and the degree of narrowing achieved [**Fig. 1** – partially complete. Being created with Elsevier illustrators]. The goal of this article is to discuss important considerations in preoperative planning, proper execution of the double-dome tip sculpting technique, unique characteristics of the individual wide tip deformities, and additional maneuvers commonly used in conjunction with the double-dome unit technique. A series of case examples are presented for clinical correlation.

## ANALYSIS

A structured and thorough preoperative analysis is the foundation of any successful rhinoplasty operation but is even more crucial for tip reconstruction. During assessment of the tip complex, the authors encourage gaining a three-dimensional understanding of the patient's anatomy by visualizing the nose from multiple angles. In the authors' practice, a complete nasal examination is performed and multiview digital photographs are taken routinely during the initial consultation. Photographs should be taken in a consistent manner and with proper lighting. Over- or underexposed pictures may obscure critical details such as tip highlight position or existing shadows. Manual palpation provides valuable information about the strength of the alar cartilages, skin thickness, and the position of the caudal septum at the anterior and posterior nasal angles. During the assessment, the surgeon should also carefully analyze the areas of tip widening to better delineate the strength, position, and convexity of the lower lateral cartilages. Bifidity and a potential obtuse interdomal angle are also important to note.

Ideal candidates for suture techniques have thin skin, strong alar cartilages, and a broad or even trapezoidal tip structure. Although these guidelines are not rigid, they do represent favorable characteristics for suture modification. If analysis of the lower alar cartilages reveals extreme

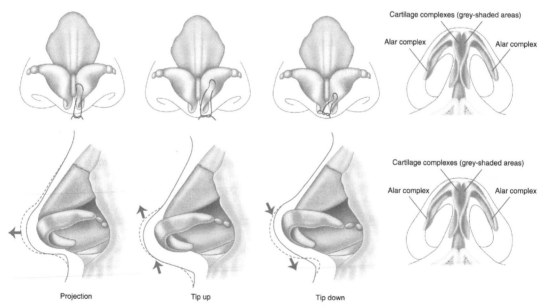

Projection          Tip up          Tip down

**Fig. 1.** Variability in suture placement in a caudal-cephalic and medial-lateral direction allows for subtle control of nasal tip projection and rotation. Understanding this, one can address an asymmetric tip using asymmetrically placed single-dome sutures. It is essential to eliminate any asymmetries at this stage of tip contouring to avoid propagating the existing deformity.

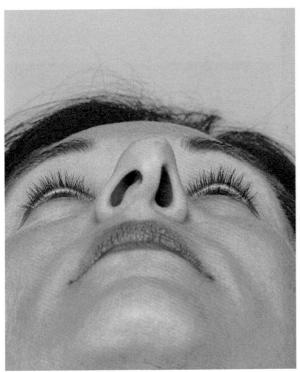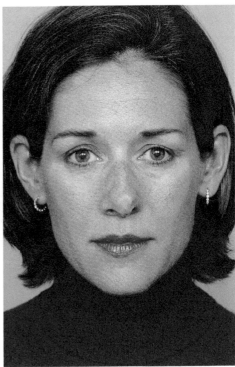

Fig. 2. Patient who has a preoperative tip deformity from congenital asymmetry in the length of the medial crura.

cephalic positioning or significant weakness, an external approach combined with alternate methods such as lateral crural repositioning or lateral crural grafts must be considered to help create the desired tip definition. Failure to recognize these characteristics may result in nasal obstruction secondary to internal recurvature of the lateral crura or delayed contour abnormalities from inadequate support.

Following manual palpation, the spatial position of the tip with respect to the individual's facial proportions is assessed. Tip projection, the degree of rotation, nasolabial angle, and dorsal height are all key elements to consider. The exact placement and orientation of an individual stitch during suture modification of the tip can especially alter rotation and projection, and therefore these characteristics must be given special consideration in surgical planning (see Fig. 1). Finally, tip asymmetries and their causes should be identified. Displacement of the caudal septum off the nasal spine, with resultant displacement of the alar cartilages, is a common cause of tip asymmetry in the posttraumatic nose. In such cases, repositioning of the caudal septum may be required in conjunction with suture techniques. In other cases, tip asymmetry may reflect congenital differences in the length or orientation of the alar cartilages (Fig. 2).

## THE FAVORABLE TIP CONTOUR

A solid understanding of nasal tip dynamics during the healing process and an awareness of the three-dimensional qualities of a favorable nasal tip contour are elements essential to attaining proficiency in the correction of the wide tip complex. As described by Toriumi,[6] a favorable tip

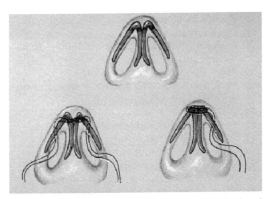

Fig. 3. Double-dome suture placement (5-0 Prolene) used to unify and stabilize the two alar complexes.

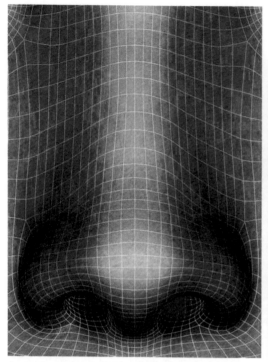
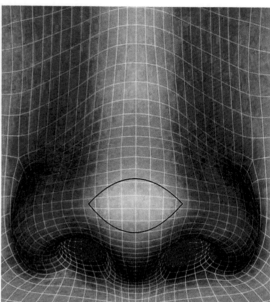

Fig. 4. The three-dimensional contour of a favorable tip illustrating a supra-alar shadow, which is effaced in the wide tip complex.

contour is characterized by a subtle shadow or concavity in the supra-alar region. In the broad tip, this concavity is often replaced by an outward convexity. The contour discrepancy is the result of a close relationship between the alar cartilage complex and the overlying skin–soft tissue envelope. In much the same way that a camping tent's shape reflects the arrangement of the underlying structural poles, the external contour of the nose is the byproduct of the configuration of its alar cartilages. Areas of cartilage that project into the skin envelope will tend to produce a highlight, whereas other areas will present as concavities or shadows. It is this

---

**Box 2**
**Surgical steps in rhinoplasty**

1. Access incisions.
2. Deliver alar cartilages.
3. Perform cephalic trim.
4. Shorten caudal septum.
5. Perform septoplasty and cartilage harvest.
6. Expose dorsum/perform profileplasty.
7. Place spreader grafts.
8. Perform single- and double-dome techniques.
9. Place alar batten or strut graft.
10. Perform single- and double-dome suturing with final modification.
11. Place columellar strut.
12. Perform medial and lateral osteotomies.
13. Place onlay or radix grafts.
14. Perform tip contour refinement with morselized cartilage or soft tissue.
15. Perform alar base narrowing.
16. Place dressings and Surgicel under the domes.

---

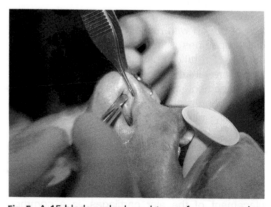

Fig. 5. A 15-blade scalpel used to perform a complete or high septal transfixion incision. The assistant uses a double-prong skin hook to retract the contralateral alar to prevent accidental injury. The complete transfixion incision can be used to deproject the nose.

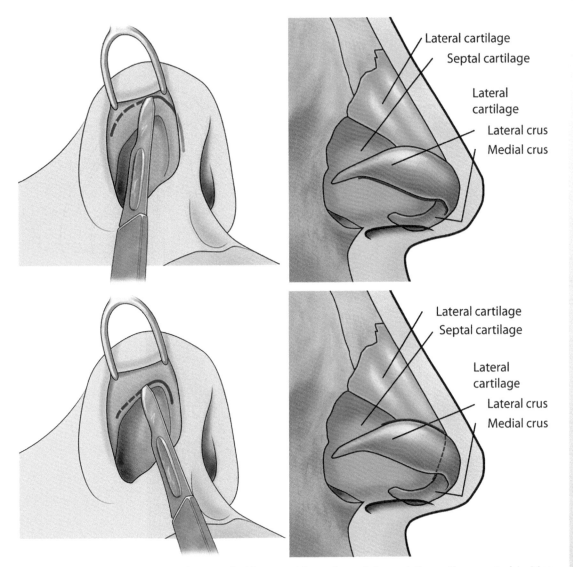

Lateral cartilage
Septal cartilage
Lateral cartilage
Lateral crus
Medial crus

**Fig. 6.** The marginal and intercartilaginous incisions used in endonasal dome delivery. The marginal incision should follow the caudal margin of the lower lateral cartilage and should not be mistaken for a rim incision.

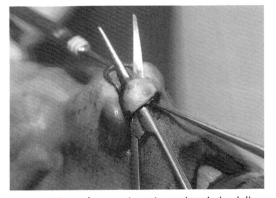

**Fig. 7.** A Metzenbaum scissor is used to help deliver and support the bipedicled chondrocutaneous flap during tip modification. The flap is often replaced into its native position after the suture is thrown and while the stitch is tied so that a "real-time" assessment of the contour effect can be performed.

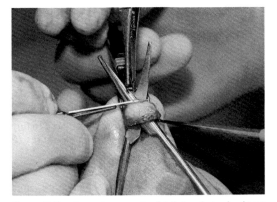

**Fig. 8.** Following placement of bilateral single-dome sutures, unilateral or bilateral "beveling" of the cephalic portion of the intermediate crura can be performed to refine the time contour and establish symmetry.

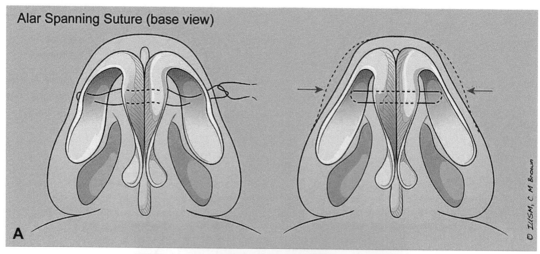

Alar Spanning Suture (base view)

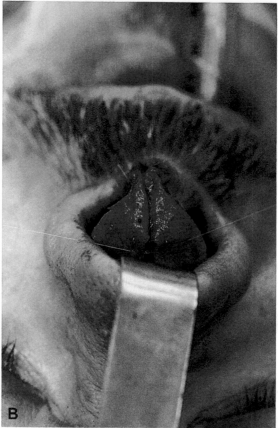

**Fig. 9.** (*A*) Alar spanning suture may be required to further narrow and eliminate excess residual tip width following placement of the single- and double-dome sutures. (*B*) Intraoperative photo of alar spanning suture placement.

subtle flow between nasal highlights and shadows that brings harmony between the individual tip subunits without abrupt contour change, and furthermore, provides a balance that restricts the observer's eye from focusing on the actual nose, and instead, on the eyes.

In a wide or broad tip, excess convexity or cephalic positioning of the lower lateral cartilages causes unfavorable width in the supra-alar region. Therefore, the conceptual goal of surgical correction of this contour abnormality is to narrow or reposition the intermediate and lateral crus into a more favorable orientation. Doing so offers control over which particular areas of the alar complex ultimately project into the skin–soft tissue envelope, and thus tip contour and shape.

## THE DOUBLE-DOME CONCEPT

In the late 1980s, McCollough and English[7] described an endonasal bidomal suture technique termed "the double-dome unit," which uses a single suture passed through the two intermediate and lateral crus to stabilize and unify the two alar complexes into a single unit (**Fig. 3**). Before placement of this bidomal suture, the tip is narrowed, and symmetry between the two alar units is attained using individual domal mattress sutures. The ultimate effect is not only a more favorable tip contour but also one that is stabilized against contractural forces (**Fig. 4**). A 15-year review of the senior author's results using the double-dome unit procedure for tip rhinoplasty shows the technique to be reliable, with consistent results and a low rate of revision.[5]

## DOUBLE-DOME TECHNIQUE

**Box 2** provides a general outline of the order in which surgical steps are performed in the authors' rhinoplasty practice. One must, however, transcend a "cookbook" approach to rhinoplasty and keep in mind that individual variations in

anatomy and expectations preclude the use of a single technique for each patient. Although the double-dome technique can be performed by way of the external or endonasal approach, the authors advocate the use of the endonasal delivery flap technique whenever possible. The endonasal approach (incorporating bilateral marginal and intercartilaginous incisions) allows for excellent visualization of tip anatomy by presenting the alar cartilages as bipedicled chondrocutaneous flaps.[5]

The delivery approach begins by making either a complete transfixion incision or a high septal transfixion, depending on existing tip projection (**Fig. 5**). Curved sharp scissors are then used to dissect up over the anterosuperior septal angle and expose the upper lateral cartilages. Next, intercartilaginous and marginal incisions are made in a standard fashion (**Fig. 6**). Thin Metzenbaum scissors are subsequently used to elevate the skin–soft tissue envelope off the underlying lower lateral cartilages. Finally, the alar domes are individually delivered with a single hook and supported with the Metzenbaum scissors. In this fashion, each dome is assessed and recontoured separately (**Fig. 7**).

The first step toward achieving improved definition is removal of the fibrofatty tissue between the domes, which will allow greater approximation of the alar cartilages. This step is particularly

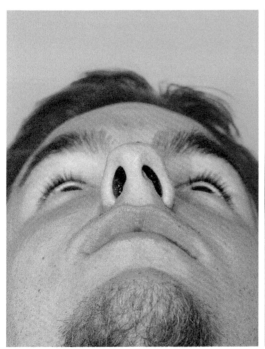
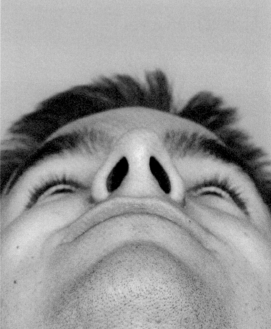

**Fig. 10.** Trapezoid tip shown on base view. Note the strong divergence of the intermediate crura.

important in cases with an obtuse interdomal angle. In appropriate situations, an intact or complete strip is subsequently performed by excising the cephalic portion of the lateral crura, which achieves volume reduction and improved supratip definition. It is essential to preserve at least a 7- to 9-mm width of cartilage. The cartilages can be repositioned in situ. In a few select cases, these steps may be all that is required. Most often, however, satisfactory tip symmetry and definition have not been achieved, and further refinement and stabilization are required.

### Single-Dome Suture: Narrowing

Once each alar dome is delivered and cephalic trimming performed, the tip can be narrowed. The vestibular skin is first separated from the undersurface of the domal cartilage, which allows more control over reshaping and prevents penetrating the vestibular mucosa with the suture needle. A 5-0 absorbable synthetic polyglycolic acid (Dexon) mattress suture is then placed at the intermediate crus and used to narrow and refine each tip-defining point.[5] By varying the orientation of the suture, tip projection and rotation

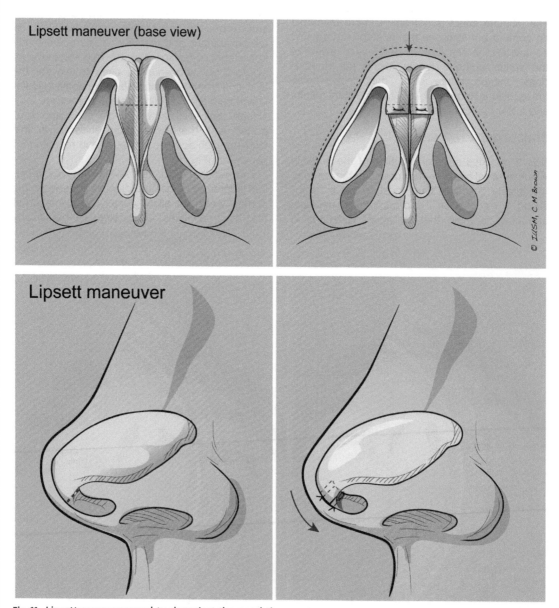

**Fig. 11.** Lipsett maneuver used to deproject the nasal tip.

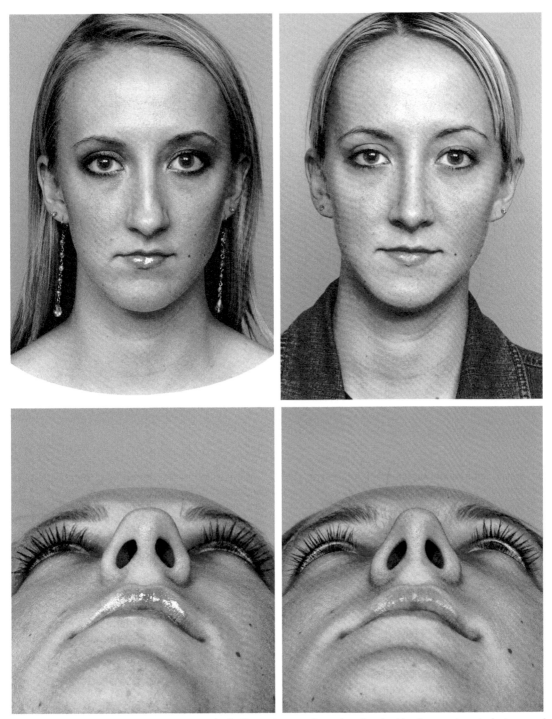

**Case example#1 (bulbous tip).** Correction of a bulbous tip complex using the double-dome suture technique and minor cephalic trim bilaterally. Tip further supported with a columellar strut.

can be modified. The knot is tightened to the point at which the proper amount of domal definition is achieved. Minor tip asymmetries created in the supratip when cinching down the suture can be further modified by "beveling" the cephalic portion of the stronger dome to match the opposite side (**Fig. 8**). Symmetry between the two domes should be established before proceeding to other tip maneuvers. Failure to do so may propagate any existing asymmetry

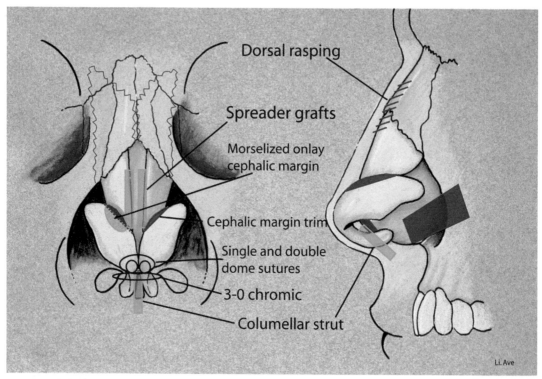

Case example #1 (bulbous tip). (continued).

### Double-Dome Suture: Unifying and Stabilizing

Following individual dome modifications, the double-dome stitch (transdomal mattress suture) is used to stabilize the individually defined domes into a single unit. This stabilization is the key for maintaining long-term results. A 5-0 clear polypropylene (Prolene) suture is placed horizontally through the lateral and intermediate crura of both domes. The amount of tension applied when cinching the knot allows control over the degree of lobule narrowing achieved. The authors advocate replacing the domes back to their native state so that a "real-time" assessment of the narrowing can be seen as the knot is tied. It is essential not to cinch the suture down completely to avoid creating a "unitip" appearance. At this point, the tip is reevaluated. Minor asymmetries can be addressed with a subtle cartilage shave or by replacing the double-dome mattress suture in a different orientation.

as each subsequent refinement maneuver is performed.

With a favorable tip contour established, an evaluation of tip support must be performed before progressing to management of the middle vault and bony pyramid. In most of the authors' cases, a columellar strut is fashioned from septal cartilage and sewn into place between the medial crura and anterior to the nasal spine. The intranasal incisions are closed with 5-0 catgut suture. In closing marginal incisions, it is important to avoid the lateral crura when suturing because it risks accidental retraction of the lateral crura and can lead to alar collapse or nostril asymmetry.

### SPECIFIC CONSIDERATIONS FOR INDIVIDUAL DEFORMITIES

Although several separate tip deformities have been grouped under the category of "wide or broad" for the simplicity of discussion, some inherent characteristics should be recognized and addressed during surgical planning and execution. Although a complete discussion of each is beyond the scope of this article, the authors present their experience in the management of the different abnormalities.

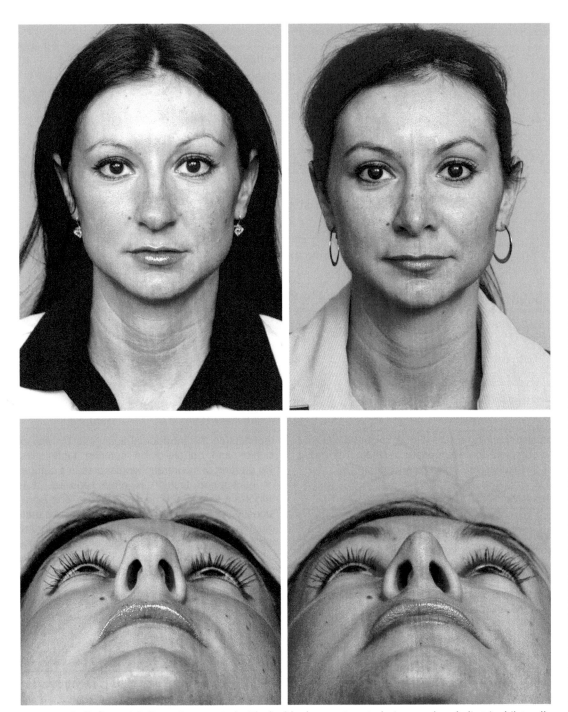

**Case example#2 (boxy tip).** Boxy tip corrected with double-dome suture technique and cephalic trim bilaterally. Tip further supported with a columellar strut.

## Bulbous Tip (Case Example #1)

The bulbous tip is an extension of a wide or broad tip in that the cartilages are more bulky and require a greater degree of individual dome refinements and narrowing. In addition to single- and double-

dome suture modification, lateral alar support is often required because the bulbous tip often has some component of cephalic malpositioning to the alar cartilages. Alar strut grafts should be considered, to flatten the excess convexity and reduce supra-alar width. Additionally, placement of

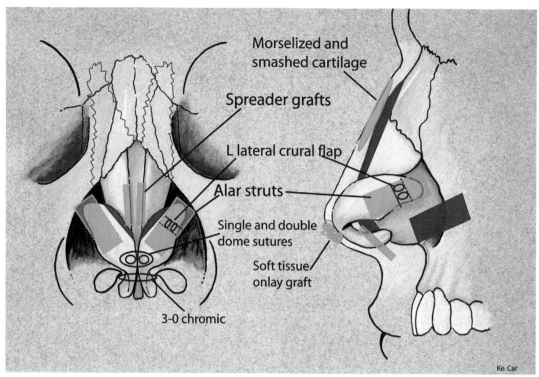

Morselized and smashed cartilage

Spreader grafts

L lateral crural flap

Alar struts

Single and double dome sutures

Soft tissue onlay graft

3-0 chromic

Ke. Car

**Case example#2 (boxy tip).** (*continued*).

an alar spanning suture (**Fig. 9**) might be required to complete the appropriate aesthetic narrowing of the excessively convex cartilages.

### Boxy Nasal Tip (Case Example #2)

The single- and double-dome suturing techniques are used to narrow the boxy tip. The boxy tip is somewhat trapezoidal but not a complete divergent intermediate crura. Weakening the strong alar cartilages is required and occasionally, camouflage in the infratip lobular area is necessary to fill in the residual bifidity.

### Trapezoid Tip

A trapezoid tip (**Fig. 10**) is a more definitive degree of the boxy tip, with marked divergence of the intermediate crura and strong alar cartilages.[8,9] It might or might not additionally involve some cephalic malposition of the alar cartilages. Surgical correction of the broad or trapezoid tip should never be performed using the cartilage splitting or transcartilaginous cephalic margin reduction technique, which would most likely result in the late development of definitive dome bossa.

Surgical correction of the broad trapezoid tip requires removal of the soft tissue between the domes and intermediate crura. One must always

reconstitute the intradomal ligaments by way of single- and double-dome suturing techniques. Tip grafting of the infratip lobular area in a sutured or nonsutured fashion is often required. It is important to support the medial crura, and occasionally the lateral ala, with a strut. Cephalic margin trim should be conservative so that further weakening of the lateral alar walls or external valve is not exacerbated, resulting in a postoperative look of recurvature of the alar cartilages. One must either reorient the cephalic position of the alar cartilages more caudally or add a caudal alar strut graft on the vestibular surface of the alar cartilage margin.

### Asymmetric or Twisted Tip (Case Example #3)

An asymmetric or twisted tip is ideally treated by a Lipsett maneuver, unilateral truncation, or by way of dome division, which can be done through the endonasal approach. If the medial crura are too twisted, however, it might be helpful to use the external columellar incision to straighten the asymmetries of the medial crura by suturing the crura together with a strut to straighten them. In such cases, the lengths of the alar cartilages are often different. The Lipsett procedure is performed posterior to the dome. A length of medial crus (1–3 mm) is excised in the intermediate crus, or incised,

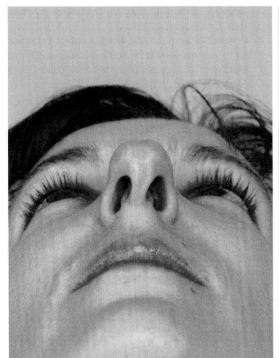
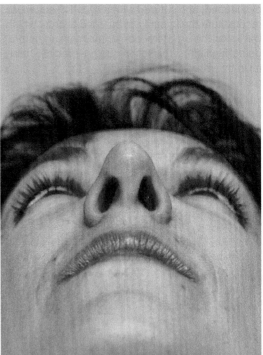

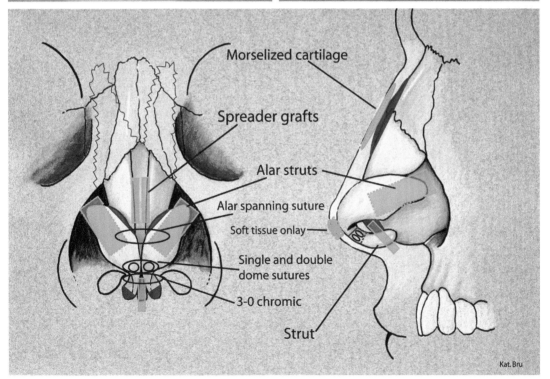

Morselized cartilage

Spreader grafts

Alar struts

Alar spanning suture

Soft tissue onlay

Single and double
dome sutures

3-0 chromic

Strut

Kat. Bru

Case example #3 (asymmetric and boxy tip). This tip complex harbors characteristics of the boxy tip and asymmetric qualities. The Lipsett maneuver (*red hatch marks of medial crura on lateral view*) used to symmetrically reposition the tip height. Alar strut grafts were required to prevent internal recurvature following placement of the double-dome and alar spanning sutures. Note the postoperative improvement in the tip lobule shape, nostril symmetry, and tip symmetry.

overlapped, and sutured with a 6-0 PDS suture, to reconstitute the integrity of the medial crus, which will lower the unilateral dome, maintaining natural domal highlights; this technique is especially helpful in thin-skinned individuals (**Fig. 11**).

## REFERENCES

1. Tebbets JB. Rethinking the logic and techniques of primary tip rhinoplasty: a perspective of the evolution of surgery of the nasal tip. Clin Plast Surg 1996;23: 245–53 [review].
2. Tardy ME Jr, Patt BS, Walter MA. Transdomal suture refinement of the nasal tip: long-term outcomes. Facial Plast Surg. 1993;9:275–84.
3. Tebbetts JB. Shaping and positioning the nasal tip without structural disruption: a new, systematic approach. Plast Reconstr Surg 1994;94:61–77.
4. Tardy ME, Brown RJ. Surgical anatomy of the nose. New York: Raven; 1990.
5. Perkins SW, Hamilton MM, MacDonald K. A successful 15 year experience in double-dome tip surgery via endonasal approach - nuances and pitfalls. Arch Facial Plast Surg 2001;3:157–64.
6. Toriumi DM. New concepts in nasal tip contouring. Arch Facial Plast Surg 2006;8:156–85.
7. McCollough EG, English JL. A new twist in nasal tip surgery: an alternative to the Goldman tip for the wide or bulbous lobule. Arch Otolaryngol 1985;111: 524–9.
8. Becker DG, Weinberger MS, Greene BA, et al. Clinical study of alar anatomy and surgery of the alar base. Arch Otolaryngol Head Nuck Surg 1997; 123(8):789–95.
9. Tardy MD Jr. Sculpturing the nasal tip. In: Tardy ME Jr, editor. Rhinoplasty - the art and science. Philadelphia: WB Saunders; 1997. p. 374–571.

# New Concepts in Nasal Tip Contouring

Dean M. Toriumi, MD[a],*, Mark A. Checcone, MD[b]

## KEYWORDS

- Nasal tip contour • Ideal nasal tip contour
- Nasal tip anatomy • Nasal tip surgery • Pinched nasal tip
- Malpositioned lateral crura

We have studied the characteristics of good-looking nasal tip structures and have come up with the concept of favorable shadowing of the nasal tip structure. After extensive study, a series of images were created that demonstrate how specific contours create highlights and shadows that are requisite for a favorable nasal tip contour. If the shadows of the nasal tip are in the proper location, then the tip will look favorable. The favorable tip contour should have a continuous high point from the domal region laterally to the alar margins bilaterally. This high point will eliminate any shadowing along the lateral margins of the domes themselves. It is this shadowing that frames the dome structure and creates the bulbous, or pinched, look to the tip structure. Ideally, one would like to see a continuous high ridge that extends from the domes to the alar lobule, which can be readily noted on the base view with no evidence of pinching around the tip area.

This tip contour can be achieved by creating a favorable width of the domes using domal suturing techniques, followed by placement of alar rim grafts. Alar rim grafts are small cartilage grafts that are placed into pockets along the caudal margin of the marginal incisions to provide support and prevent pinching around the dome structure.

Some patients may have cephalic orientation of the lateral crura, which will not allow favorable shadowing of the tip structure. Correction may require repositioning of the lateral crura into a caudally positioned pocket. This maneuver will help create more favorable shadowing around the nasal tip.

Contouring the nasal tip requires a clear understanding of what looks normal and which methods should be used to attain that contour. Simply narrowing the nasal tip is not sufficient because these maneuvers may create abnormal shadowing and the pinched-tip look. The surgeon must learn to visualize the nasal tip from a three-dimensional perspective, with emphasis on contours affecting shadowing. Proper use of suturing and repositioning techniques in combination with cartilage grafting will help create favorable, natural-appearing tip contours. The focus needs to be more on reorienting shadowing around the nasal tip and less on simply narrowing the nasal tip.

The nasal tip, or lower third of the nose as a whole, deserves special attention for its particular complexities, both aesthetically and functionally. The nasal tip, as a proper subunit, and its adjoining subunits (columella, facets, and alae) compose the lower third of the nose. This area is physiologically dynamic because it moves with inspiration, expiration, and facial expression. It functions as a powerful shock absorber for facial trauma and a delicate icon of facial beauty. Its central position on a person's face makes it impossible to ignore when it is disharmonious with other facial contours; however, when appropriately formed, it nearly disappears as attention is drawn more to a person's eyes and other distinguishing

[a] Division of Facial Plastic and Reconstructive Surgery, Department of Otolaryngology–Head and Neck Surgery, University of Illinois Chicago, 1855 W. Taylor Street, Room 2.42 (MC 648), Chicago, IL 60612-7244, USA
[b] Department of Otolaryngology–Head and Neck Surgery, Washington University in St. Louis School of Medicine, St. Louis, MO, USA
* Corresponding author.
*E-mail address:* dtoriumi@uic.edu (D.M. Toriumi).

Facial Plast Surg Clin N Am 17 (2009) 55–90
doi:10.1016/j.fsc.2008.10.001

facial features. The rhinoplasty surgeon's goal is to shape the nose in a manner that creates harmony with the entire face. Unlike the upper and middle two thirds of the nose, the lower third of the nose continues to present the greatest challenge when setting out to achieve this task.

The difficulty of shaping the tip during rhinoplasty stems in part from the three-dimensional complexities of this structure. When viewed from the front, the lower third of the nose is an intricate array of highlights and shadows, which are a product of the many curvilinear surface transitions occurring in three dimensions: vertically, horizontally, and anteroposteriorly. Altering the profile is a two-dimensional task focused on aligning the supratip to meet a straight dorsal profile and transitioning the infratip and columella to create an appropriate nasolabial angle. The three-dimensional concept of tip contouring is more complex than the two-dimensional concept of profile alignment from the viewpoint of nasal analysis and surgical technique. Evidence of this complexity is the frequent presentation of secondary rhinoplasty patients who demonstrate pinched or asymmetric middle nasal vaults, supra-alar pinching of the nasal sidewall, or unnaturally pointed or asymmetric tips. An otherwise good rhinoplasty outcome with an attractive profile is compromised by even the slightest concavity or asymmetry in the tip, which results in unnaturally positioned shadows that detract from the person's appearance on frontal view. The profile view is much more forgiving and can tolerate dorsum-to-tip differences of 2 to 3 mm while still appearing appropriate. Most people, including patients on self-inspection in a mirror, scrutinize the frontal view and not the profile, to determine a satisfactory result. It is also the frontal view that is more susceptible to ongoing contour changes as a result of wound contracture over time. Although the profile tends to stabilize early in the healing process, the frontal view sees dramatic changes over the course of many years.

The purpose of this article is to present the reader with the necessary knowledge and skills to reshape the lower third of the nose and to create a natural-appearing tip with longevity. Controlling tip shape requires a comprehensive execution of nasal tip aesthetic analysis, careful consideration of the underlying anatomic structures, and recognition of the significant contractile forces caused by wound healing for many years following surgery. Failure to recognize these key elements results in several common iatrogenic nasal tip deformities, which are discussed in more detail.

In contrast to traditional tip-narrowing methods, the techniques presented here provide complimentary support to strengthen the underlying nasal skeleton in a manner that naturally contours the external nasal tip yet resists the internal forces of contracture over the patient's lifetime of healing.

## NASAL ANALYSIS

Preoperative nasal analysis must consist of a careful study of external contour anomalies, correlation with anatomic structural support, and thoughtful consideration of the ultimate ideal contour for that particular patient. It is the integration of these three important goals that distinguishes a good outcome from a satisfactory one. First, creating an appropriate nasal tip requires a proper interpretation of the various highlights and shadows that form on the exterior nasal surface as a result of light reflection and refraction against the convex and concave surfaces that define the external appearance. During an initial patient consultation, it is important to obtain accurate clinical photographs. Ideally, photographs should be taken with a single light source and again with two light sources to correctly identify and document all preexisting contour depressions or asymmetries. These photographs are of particular value for the frontal view where certain contours appear different, depending on how light reflects and shadows are cast (**Fig. 1**). For single-light photography, the light is positioned slightly

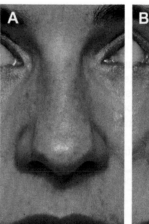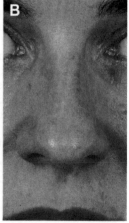

**Fig. 1.** The same patient is photographed twice before any procedures. (*A*) This photograph was taken with a single flash. More shadowing is seen around the tip, and the bulbous appearance looks more dramatic when compared with *B*. (*B*) This photograph was taken with two flashes. Notice how fewer shadows are cast laterally and that the tip appears less bulbous than in *A*.

above the camera, along the centerline. When photographing with two lights, each is placed in the same horizontal plane slightly above the patient's face and equidistant from the subject along a line 45° from center. This constant lighting setup makes external contour analysis consistent among patients and reproducible on the same patient postoperatively. Next, the underlying nasal skeleton and soft tissue covering that make up the anatomic supporting structures should be studied in the context of their position, size, and shape. Surgical modification of any of these elements will have an effect on external contours. Finally, it is necessary for the self-improving rhinoplasty surgeon to constantly reexamine the socially and culturally acceptable "ideal" nasal form. The success of rhinoplasty is judged not by one view but by all six clinical views. The exponentially more difficult view to perfect is the frontal view and thus it will remain the focus of this article.

## Analyzing External Contours

Nasal contours on lateral view are defined by the sharp contrast between the nasal skin and a contrasting colored background. The frontal view has a more subtle contour that is defined by the less obvious contrasts between highlights of light reflecting off convex surfaces and shadows created by refracted light on concave areas. The most prominent light reflexes appear along the most anteriorly positioned convexities like the nasal tip, dorsum, and glabella. Considering the normal anatomy of the human face, the ideal frontal nasal silhouette has a slight hourglass appearance from the eyebrows to the nasal tip.[1] Tardy[2] first coined this "the brow–tip aesthetic line," which he described as a continuous curvilinear line extending from the medial brow to the nasal tip, with the narrowest part along the nasal vault and two divergent concave curves superiorly and inferiorly (**Fig. 2**). Any disruption to this line draws attention in an unfavorable way.

Several common deformities can disrupt the brow–tip aesthetic line. Any asymmetries of the supraorbital rims, glabella, radix, bony dorsum, cartilaginous dorsum, or tip can alter this contour. Focusing on the tip for the purposes of this article, disruption of the frontal silhouette can occur as a result of trauma, iatrogenic deformity, or preexisting anatomic anomalies. An example of the last, tip bulbosity, is the result of excessive supratip fullness that disrupts the brow–tip aesthetic line. Rather than gracefully transitioning from the concave line along the upper two thirds to a convex lower third, the bulbous tip creates a sudden divergence that sharply breaks the curvature of the

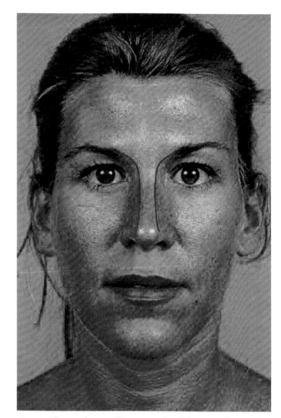

**Fig. 2.** The red, curvilinear, paired lines indicate the brow–tip aesthetic line. When viewed on frontal view, an outline of the highlights cast on the nose should form a subtle hourglass shape. Starting superiorly at the medial brow, the line curves along a concave path following the supraorbital rim to join the radix or nasal root, then gradually narrows to form a relatively straight line along the bony and cartilaginous dorsum, before gracefully diverging outward to outline a slightly wider nasal supratip and fading laterally along a confluent alar-tip lobule. (*From* Toriumi DM. New concepts in nasal tip contouring. Arch Facial Plast Surg 2006;8:156–185; with permission. Copyright © 2006, American Medical Association. All rights reserved.)

brow–tip aesthetic line (**Fig. 3**). The underlying causes of the bulbous tip are discussed more in the next section. Iatrogenically created tip deformities are a common occurrence and often mimic the patient's unfavorable bulbous tip appearance. Patients frequently complain about having a "ball on my tip" that never really improved even after rhinoplasty surgery. Careful analysis of their nasal contours, however, reveals that the "ball-like" appearance is not the result of an untreated bulbous tip. Rather, the tip is often overly narrowed to create an unnatural shadow between the supratip

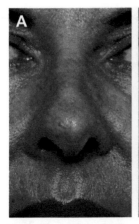
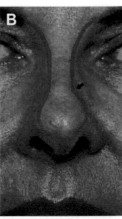

**Fig. 3.** The bulbous tip has supratip fullness that disrupts the brow–tip aesthetic line. (*A*) Note the dark shadows around the supratip, which is more apparent on the patient's left side. (*B*) The brow–tip aesthetic lines are superimposed over the same photograph approximating the line created by the transition from nasal highlights to shadows. An arrow indicates the unnatural break created in the brow–tip aesthetic line by a laterally divergent bulbous supratip highlight.

lobule and the alar lobule. On frontal view, the ball-shaped tip gets its appearance from obscure dome highlights surrounded by improperly placed shadows on either ala (**Fig. 4**), which effectively circumscribe the tip with shadows from the supratip break above, the infratip break below, and the

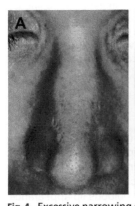
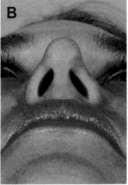

**Fig. 4.** Excessive narrowing or pinching of the nasal tip can result in unfavorable shadows or an unnatural demarcation between the tip lobule and alar lobules. (*A*) Note the ball-shaped tip that is created by a narrow tip highlight completely circumscribed by shadows. (*B*) The pinched tip is created by narrowing of the medial alae, resulting in concaved lateral alar walls that make the tip look like a constricted ball.

lateral alae on the left and right. The base view provides structural evidence of the cause of these lateral shadows. The alar margins collapse medially, creating a concavity where a straight or slightly convex alar margin should exist. The net effect is a pinched lateral alar wall that creates an overly rounded tip that is analogous to a constricted ball.

### Analyzing Anatomic Support

Features of a naturally formed tip include appropriate skin thickness, adequate fibrofatty tissue volume, and proper cartilaginous support. Details about techniques that manipulate these tissues are discussed later. However, it is necessary to first understand how the underlying anatomy of a naturally beautiful nose contributes to the nasal tip contour before one can manipulate these tissues in an attempt to transform a flawed nasal tip contour into one that is appropriately shaped.

Skin thickness assessment is helpful before surgery to determine how well the external cover will redrape over the underlying bone, cartilage, and subcutaneous tissue in a way that creates graceful contours. Fibrofatty tissue provides most of the volume in both alar lobules and, to a smaller degree, the nasal tip. Medium-thickness skin is the most ideal. Skin that is excessively thick masks the underlying structures, leading to decreased definition or refinement. Overly thinned skin has the reverse effect, where too much detail of the underlying structures is seen and sharp angulations or step-offs of bone and cartilage become too apparent. Proper evaluation of the skin thickness and fibrofatty tissue volume during preoperative consultation is imperative for the benefit of the surgeon planning surgery and, more importantly, for the benefit of the patient, who should be appropriately counseled about expectations following surgery.

Critical to both the form and function of the nasal tip, the upper and lower lateral cartilages require adequate strength, shape or form, and position. The upper lateral cartilages span a varying degree of vertical height, depending on the patient. The dorsal length of the nose is made up of contributions from the nasal bones and the upper lateral cartilages. The dorsal width is maintained to create a uniform brow–tip aesthetic line when the upper lateral cartilages are of sufficient strength to resist pinching. Favorable anatomic configuration includes longer nasal bones, shorter upper lateral cartilages, and uniform bony and cartilaginous widths.

The lower lateral cartilages are the main support structure for the nasal tip and each individual component influences the exterior form. Starting with the medial aspect of the lower lateral carti-lages, the footplates and the adjacent nasal spine create the underlying base or pedestal of the nose. Noses with long, strong medial crura and medial crural footplates that extend down to the nasal spine have excellent support and will tend not to lose projection postoperatively (**Fig. 5**A). A common example of nasal base weakness can be found in noses where the medial crura is of inadequate length and the footplates appear to be floating at the midcolumella rather than extending completely down to the nasal spine (**Fig. 5**B). This structural insufficiency is not only visible but also palpable by manually depressing the tip posteriorly to feel the weakness in the nasal base. The transition from medial crus to intermediate crus creates a subtle lateral flare that contributes to the soft tissue facet on base view and defines the infratip lobular double break point on the lateral and oblique views. The domes are the most projecting point of the lower lateral cartilages where the intermediate crura sharply bend to form the lateral crura. The domal angle is formed by the angle between a line drawn through the intermediate crus and one drawn through the lateral crus (**Fig. 6**). The lateral crus projects superolaterally to support the lower nasal sidewall and to provide external nasal valve patency on inspiration.

The contribution of the domes and lateral crura to tip shape is an advanced concept that requires careful examination of each cartilage's size, shape, angulation, position, and orientation. In many favorably contoured tips, the caudal margin of the lateral crus lies in nearly the same horizontal plane as the cephalic margin, which creates a defined lateral alar ridge between the tip and alar lobules and, furthermore, orients the cartilage in a more supportive configuration such that the width of the lateral crus (not thickness) resists the bulk of the collapsing forces of inspiration and manual pinching on the external valve (**Fig. 7**). The cephalic margin of the lateral crus is not dramatically, but only slightly, more superior to the inferior margin of the lateral crus. Stated another way, if a horizontal plane is drawn through the patient's vertical axis and intersects a sagittal cross-sectional area of the lateral crus at its midpoint, the cephalic margin of the lateral crus lies only slightly above (superior to) the caudal margin (**Fig. 8**). The superior position of the cephalic margin over an inferior position of the caudal margin seems obvious. However, tip shape can be significantly affected by even minor deviations from this ideal positioning of the lateral crura. When a greater vertical discrepancy exists between these margins, both structure and cosmesis may be negatively impacted.

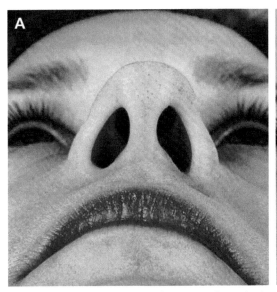
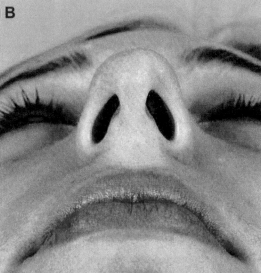

**Fig. 5.** The base view provides information about the length and strength of the medial crura, which helps assess the stability of the nasal base. (*A*) This patient, who has long, strong medial crura that extend to the nasal spine, will be less likely to lose tip projection postoperatively. (*B*) This patient, who has short medial crura that do not completely extend down to the nasal spine, has flaring footplates at the midcolumella that create an unnaturally wide base and narrow nostrils.

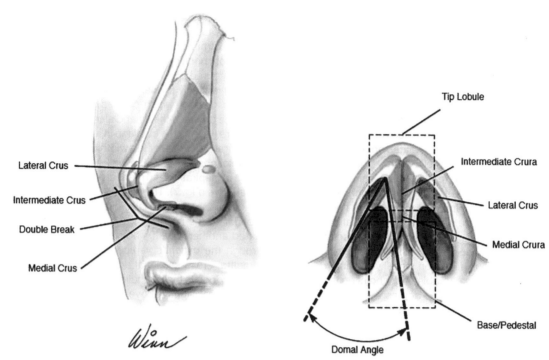

**Fig. 6.** The key structural components of the nasal tip. Note the normal divergence of the intermediate crura that is responsible for the columellar-lobular angle or double break. On base view, the foundation of the tip contains the base or pedestal, which is composed of the nasal spine and medial crural footplates. The tip lobule consists of the intermediate crura, domes, and medial portions of the lateral crura. A sufficiently wide domal angle establishes the nostril opening and supports the lateral alar wall.

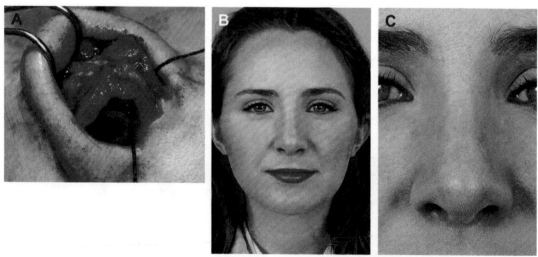

**Fig. 7.** To maximize support of the alar margin, the caudal margin of the lateral crura should lie near the same level as the cephalic margin of the lateral crura. (*A*) This patient had cephalic positioning of the lateral crura. The lateral crura were dissected from the vestibular skin, and a lateral crural strut graft was sutured to the undersurface of the lateral crura. Note how the caudal margin of the lateral crura lies near the same level as the cephalic margin of the lateral crura. (*B*) Postoperative frontal view of this patient shows a natural-appearing nasal tip with normal contours. The width of the nose fits with the round shape of her face. (*C*) This close-up postoperative frontal view of the same patient shows how the alar margins are well supported, with a good transition from tip to alar lobule. Shadowing occurs in the supratip that transitions into the supra-alar groove. The horizontal orientation of the tip is represented by the two light reflexes over the dome structures and is highlighted by the two light sources directed at 45° off midline. (*From* Toriumi DM. New concepts in nasal tip contouring. Arch Facial Plast Surg 2006;8:156–185; with permission. Copyright © 2006, American Medical Association. All rights reserved.)

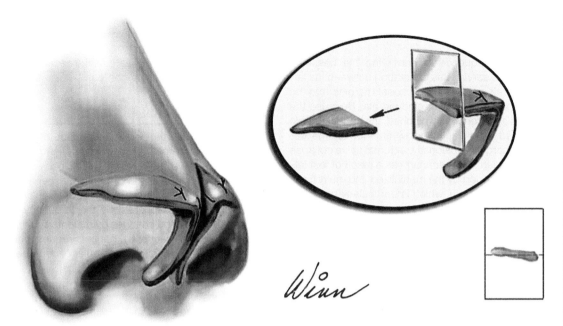

**Fig. 8.** To provide good support to the alar margin, it is preferable to have the caudal margin of the lateral crura lie in a horizontal plane that is only slightly inferior to that of the cephalic margin of the lateral crura. In the oval inset, a sagittal cross-section through a favorably orientated lateral crus illustrates how the caudal margin of the lateral crura lies in nearly the same horizontal plane (*orange dashed line*) as the cephalic margin. The sagittal plane is pictured in the lower right corner, with an orange dashed line representing a horizontal plane through the patient's vertical axis. The cephalic margin of the lateral crus is only slightly superior to the caudal margin.

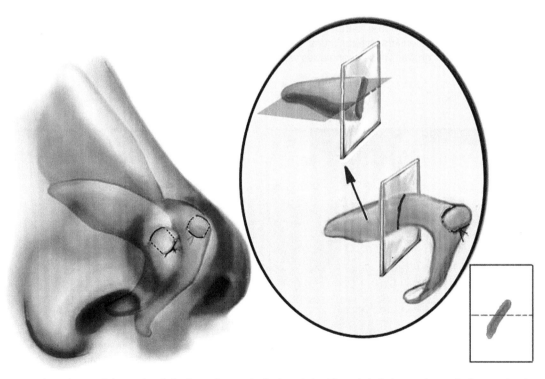

**Fig. 9.** When the caudal margin of the lateral crura is displaced significantly inferior to the cephalic margin, the alar lobule may lose support, giving the tip a pinched appearance. Pictured inside the oval inset, a cross-section through the lateral crus illustrates the unfavorable angulation of the cartilage with the caudal margin much more inferior to the cephalic margin with respect to the horizontal plane indicated in orange. In the lower right corner, a sagittal plane through the lateral crus demonstrates how the cephalic margin of the crus is much more superior (above the horizontal orange dashed line) than the inferiorly positioned caudal margin.

The consequence of narrowing the nasal tip without preserving this orientation between the lateral crura's cephalic and caudal margins may be an amorphous tip with pinched ala. Because the domes are excessively pinched, the caudal margin is forced significantly below (inferior to) the cephalic margin. Additionally, external valve collapse may be seen in this scenario as a result of lost lateral wall support by the medialized and malrotated lateral crus (Fig. 9), which is particularly problematic when the caudal margin was close to the level of the cephalic margin preoperatively. This change creates a smaller tip structure to support the same-sized skin envelope. On frontal view, an unnatural shadow separates the tip lobule from the alae where one would expect a continuous ridge of highlight (Fig. 10). The end result of this improperly narrowed tip is an overly medialized lateral crus, an unnaturally rotated caudal margin inferiorly, and an external contour that may exhibit excessive shadowing between the tip and the alae, which disrupts the smooth transition that should exist there. It is not uncommon to see this type of lower lateral cartilage deformity in some primary rhinoplasty patients. Their native cartilages can be shaped and positioned in this disadvantageous posture. Corrective measures in these cases include a combination of dome sutures, lateral crus repositioning maneuvers, lateral crural strut grafts, and alar rim grafts. These techniques are discussed in greater detail later in the section entitled, "Controlling nasal tip contour."

## Ideal Nasal Tip Contour

It is unlikely that the evasive concept of ideal beauty will be ever pinned down and defined in explicit terms. However, the concept of an ideal nasal contour within a range of socially acceptable desirability is probably within reach. Cultural consensus certainly is apparent by the frequency of commonly requested changes by patients seeking rhinoplasty. Most frequently, patients request narrower, more refined tips and complain about their pre-existing wide bases or bulbous tips.

Other investigators have formulated geometric descriptions of the ideal tip shape. Sheen and Sheen[1] modeled the ideal tip with two equilateral geodesic triangles, whose common bases are formed by a curved line drawn horizontally across the tip to connect points lying at each domal highlight. They noted that the most projecting point of the tip should lie along the apogee of the curved line between the domes. They also defined the intercrural distance as the distance between the domes. Daniel[3] noted an angle of dome definition along the domal junction line that included a convex segment along the lateral dome and a concave segment at the adjoining medial portion of the lateral crus. Based on this description, many

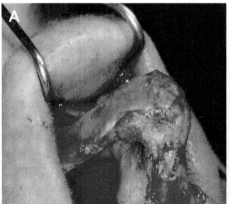
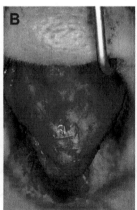
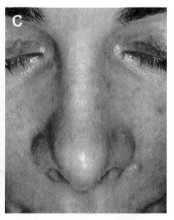

Fig. 10. In this patient, the dome-suturing method created an abnormal relationship between the caudal and cephalic margins of the lateral crura. (A) Intraoperative view of the cartilages reveals that the caudal margin of the lateral crus is significantly inferior to the cephalic margin of the lateral crus. (B) From the frontal view, one can see the dome sutures that are pinching the domes. This view demonstrates the extent of descent of the caudal margin of the lateral crura below the cephalic margin. (C) The frontal view of this patient demonstrates the isolation of the tip lobule and the pinched appearance of the nasal tip. Demarcation of the nasal tip is obvious and shadows between the tip and alar lobules are visible. The descent of the caudal margin of the lateral crura resulted in loss of support of the alar margin. Additionally, the pinched cartilage structure is too small for this patient's skin envelope, leaving the amorphous tip contour.

tip-refining techniques have sought to convert a convex lateral crus into one that is more concave. Accentuating such a concavity in an extreme manner can pinch the tip and create an unattractive demarcation between the tip lobule and the alar lobule similar to the constricted ball described earlier.

The senior author (DMT) studied numerous aesthetically pleasing nasal tips from models in fashion magazines to establish a reference for natural-looking, attractive noses that contemporary society views favorably. Attractive tips are not always narrower, but have favorable placement of light reflection and shadowing to create a more graceful transition from tip lobule to alar lobules. Even broad noses, which were included in the magazines and thus considered equally attractive, demonstrated appropriate lighting transitions between alar-tip lobules. In an effort to communicate concepts of favorable nasal tip contour, the senior author designed a series of images to demonstrate how specific contours create highlights and shadows that impart a three-dimensional perspective (**Figs. 11–14**). This article attempts to show the relationship between anatomic structure and the resulting external form. By integrating the lessons learned during almost 20 years of surgical experience, the senior author is able to impart to the reader several strategies to correctly describe natural contours, recognize the underlying causes of unnatural contours, and effectively identify techniques that will favorably manipulate the nasal tip.

On frontal view, the aesthetically pleasing nasal tip possesses some width in a horizontal plane that extends in continuity into the alar margin, forming a dome highlight outlined by two curved opposing lines (see **Fig. 11**). This horizontally oriented tip highlight represents the horizontal positioning of the domes of the lower lateral cartilages or their structural equivalent (ie, when an onlay, cap, or shield graft is present). The lateral margins of the

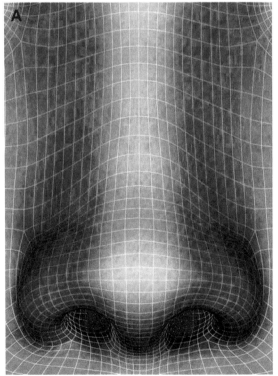
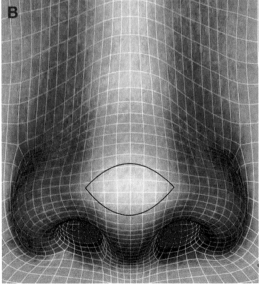

**Fig. 11.** Favorable nasal tip contour has a horizontal orientation, with a shadow in the supratip area that continues into the supra-alar regions. (*A*) The transition from the tip lobule to the alar lobule is smooth, without a line of demarcation. The tip-defining points are seen as a horizontally oriented highlight with shadows above and below. (*B*) Two horizontally oriented, opposing curved lines outline the tip highlight. The lateral extent of the highlight should continue into an elevated ridge that passes in continuity with the curvilinear contour of the alar lobule.

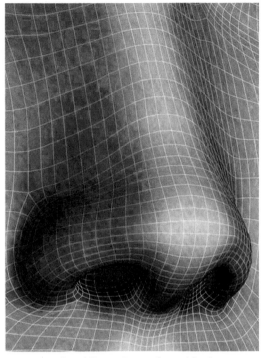

Fig. 12. On the oblique view, a favorable tip contour should demonstrate a subtle supratip break shadow that continues into the supra-alar groove. These shadows represent narrowing as the tip transitions into the supratip and middle nasal vault. The soft tissue triangles or facets should be subtle, casting only an attenuated shadow.

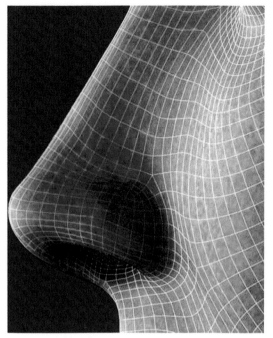

Fig. 14. On the lateral view, the tip projects above the dorsum with a supratip break. Most surgically untreated noses have a slightly more cephalic supratip break, preserving a rounder nasal tip. The double break is soft, with a subtle shadow at the soft tissue triangle. A more refined tip is created by lowering the position of the supratip break.

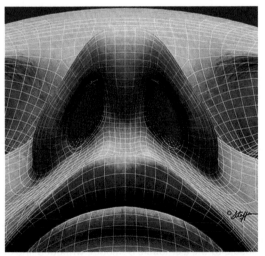

Fig. 13. The base view shows a triangular shape with no notching between the tip lobule and the alar lobule. Note the horizontal component of the nasal tip, with a defined width set by the position of the domes.

tip highlight should continue laterally as an elevated ridge that passes in continuity with the curvilinear contour of the alar lobule (see **Fig. 11B**). This horizontally oriented tip highlight is best visualized with a single midline light source directed toward the patient. If two light sources are present, then one will see two light reflexes approximating the dome highlights oriented horizontally. The exact configuration of this highlight varies among patients but in most women it is 8 mm in width, with a range of 6 to 14 mm.[3] These dimensions are slightly increased in men and in non-Caucasian patients who have thicker skin.

Equally important, a subtle shadow exists in the supratip region that continues laterally into the left and right supra-alar grooves, representing a narrowing effect cephalic to the nasal tip. Best seen on the oblique view, the shadows that are cast along the supra-alar groove and supratip are contrasted by a whiter band of highlight located along the elevated alar margin ridge and horizontal tip highlights (see **Fig. 12**). The depth of the supratip shadow correlates with the severity of the supratip break. In other words, a darker shadow is cast in the supratip area if the tip is offset from the dorsum by a greater distance (more severe supratip break). The height of the supratip shadow on the frontal view correlates with the vertical position of the supratip break on the lateral view. A poorly defined supratip break, in most unoperated noses, is typically the result of a higher-than-ideal break point on the lateral view. Typically, this problem is corrected by performing a cephalic trim of the lateral crura to reduce the vertical height of the domes, which moves the supratip break inferiorly to create a more refined tip.

On the base view, the nose should have a rounded triangular shape absent of any lateral alar wall pinching or concavity between the tip and alar lobules (see **Fig. 13**). A straight or slightly convex alar sidewall extending from tip lobule to alar lobule ensures a smooth transition between both structures on the frontal view. The soft tissue triangles or facets should have soft contour lines that fade gradually to join the columella centrally and the nostril rims laterally. The infratip lobule contour is also critical to creating a natural-looking nose. It is created by the junction between the columella and the tip lobule. This junction is marked by the infratip highlight contrasted against a shadowed columella situated more posteriorly and can be seen on oblique and base views (see **Figs. 12, 13**). The previously reported analogy of a gull in flight has been used to describe this contour formed by the infratip lobule as the alar margins meet the columella when viewed from the front.[2-5]

On lateral view, the nasal tip should have a smooth curvilinear shape with no sharp angular breaks except for the nasolabial angle. However, two important subtle contour breaks create a more refined tip and are best seen on the lateral view. Cephalically, a fluid supratip break should be apparent, which is a small indentation of the external skin surface created by a separation between the most projecting point of the domes and a more posteriorly positioned anterior septal angle (see **Fig. 14**). The second key break point, the double break or columellar-lobular angle, is seen caudal to the tip lobule (**Fig. 15**). The contour of the tip between these two break points is a consistently convex contour with a gradually variable radius of curvature, which enables different individuals to exhibit many variations of specific tip shape; however, they all fall into a common range of uniformly rounded curves absent of any sharp corners, concavities, or sudden changes in the radius of curve.

The creation or manipulation of these particular break points illustrates the importance of integrating the skills necessary to diagnose contour deformities, reposition anatomic structures, and reach the goal of an ideal nasal tip contour. The supratip break is seen as an attenuated supratip shadow on the frontal and oblique views (see **Figs. 11, 12**). The desired distance that the surgeon aims to set between the domes and septum to create the supratip break is dependent on the patient's skin thickness. Because the skin drapes over this intentional cartilaginous contour break, a thicker external cover requires a greater distance between septum and domes, whereas a thinner dermal cover may reveal a step-off unless that distance of separation is reduced. A safe guide is to allow an 8- to 10-mm distance between the leading point of the domes and the anterior septal angle for thick skin, and about a 6- to 8-mm distance for thin skin.[6,7] The reader should be forewarned that these distances are based on a tip position that will not change significantly postoperatively. If the base of the tip is not sufficiently stable, tip projection will be lost postoperatively. In the case of a modest loss of tip projection, the supratip break may be eliminated; however, extensive loss of tip projection may result in supratip fullness (pollybeak deformity). Some surgeons purposefully create a pronounced supratip break in anticipation of some inevitable postoperative loss of tip projection. This approach can leave an unpredictable variance in the prominence of the supratip break from patient to patient. It is preferable to first stabilize the nasal base effectively and then establish tip projection reliably for more consistent outcomes. Similar attention to the infratip is required to safeguard against iatrogenic disruption of the columellar-lobular angle or double break point. It is preserved by maintaining the normal divergence of the intermediate crura (see **Fig. 15**).[1,3] Subtle control of the double break can be achieved by using cartilage grafts placed around the dome structure to either soften a sharply angled double break or create a flattened one. Soft, bruised cartilage placed caudally to the intermediate crura adds bulk and can blunt a pronounced columellar-lobular angle. Thick or double-layered shield grafts, or those that are long and stiff, risk obliterating the double break and may create a flat appearance to the infratip lobule on lateral view.[8] Therefore, tip grafts must be slightly curved, with their concave surface placed against the underlying cartilage, and should be carved to match the natural divergence of the intermediate crura to preserve an appropriate double break.

## OPERATIVE TECHNIQUE

If used properly, most nasal tip techniques can create a nasal tip that looks natural. It is when techniques are overdone that deformity occurs. Some methods of nasal tip surgery deliver more

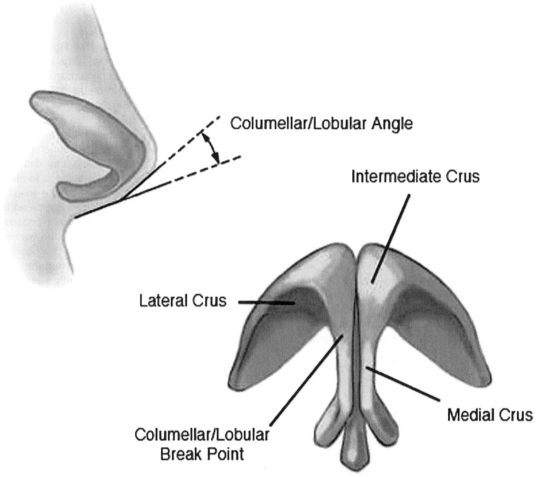

**Fig. 15.** The normal divergence of the intermediate crura creates the columellar-lobular angle or double break. For clarity of illustration, the columellar-lobular angle and divergence between the intermediate crura have been exaggerated. The distance between the domes and the divergence of the intermediate crura can be decreased to create a favorable tip contour. One should avoid suturing the intermediate crura together to avoid blunting the columellar-lobular angle.

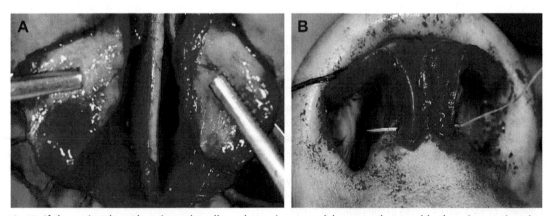

**Fig. 16.** If the patient has a hanging columella and prominent caudal septum that would otherwise require trimming, the surgeon can set the medial crura back on the midline caudal septum. (*A*) Dissection between the medial crura with elevation of bilateral mucoperichondrial flaps and exposure of the septum. (*B*) The caudal septum is too long, so the medial crura are sutured to the caudal septum with 4-0 plain catgut suture on a straight septal needle. Note that the caudal septum is sutured between the medial crura to stabilize the base of the nose. The fixation sutures are placed along the cephalic margin of the medial crura to avoid retraction of the columella. Special care is taken to create symmetry of the tip structures.

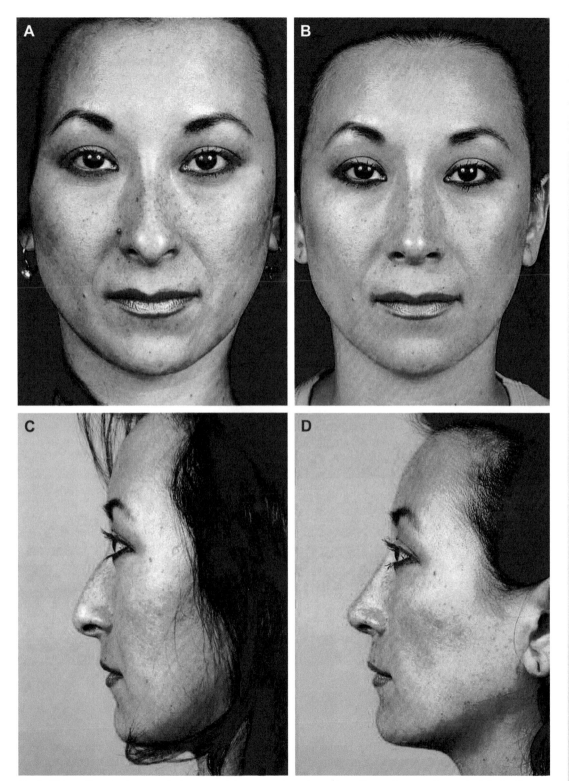

Fig. 17. This patient had an overly long caudal septum, hanging columella, and a prominent tip lobule. She underwent dissection between her medial crura with elevation of bilateral mucoperichondrial flaps. The medial crura were sutured to the overly long midline caudal septum to elevate her tip lobule and correct the hanging columella. She also underwent placement of lateral crural strut grafts and dome sutures to correct the bulbous tip. *A, C, E,* and *G* are preoperative views; *B, D, F,* and *H* are 2-year postoperative views. (*From* Toriumi DM. New concepts in nasal tip contouring. Arch Facial Plast Surg 2006;8:156–185; with permission. Copyright © 2006, American Medical Association. All rights reserved.)

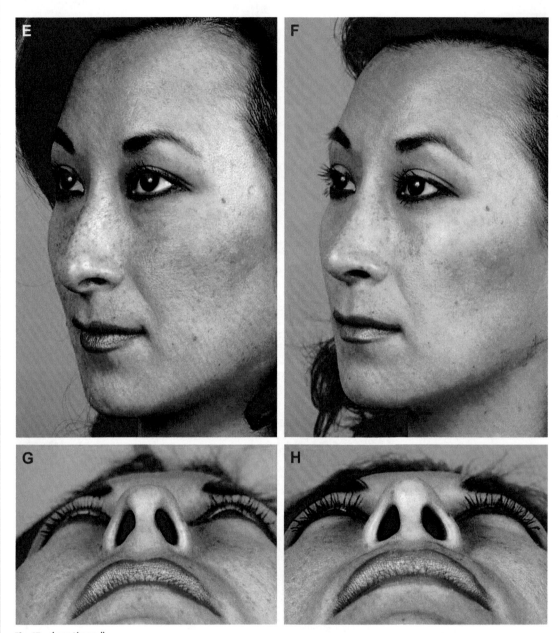

**Fig. 17.** (*continued*).

predictable results than others. The techniques described herein are reliable and versatile methods for creating a structurally stable, natural-looking nasal tip.

### Stabilizing the Nasal Base

A mandatory prerequisite to the execution of any nasal tip contouring techniques is proper stabilization of the base or pedestal of the nose (see **Fig. 6**).[4,8,9] Stabilizing the base ensures a solid foundation for the lower third of the nose, and is critical to avoid postoperative loss of nasal tip projection. Base stabilization also establishes the nasolabial angle and alar-columellar relationship. Many surgeons spend most of their time altering the region of the domes and do not correct deficiencies of the base of the nose, resulting in unpredictable losses of tip projection postoperatively. Thus, due diligence is necessary to examine base stability during preoperative nasal analysis.

If the base is well supported by the medial crura and the alar-columellar relationship does not require modification, a sutured-in-place columellar strut can stabilize the base effectively.[8] This graft is placed between the medial crura after dissecting the intercrural soft tissue attachments to create a narrow pocket. A more common scenario is that the patient requires alteration of the tip projection, the alar-columellar relationship, and the nasolabial angle. Several reliable and versatile methods can achieve these goals during the act of stabilizing the base. Three frequently used techniques include suturing the medial crura to an overly long caudal septum, using a caudal extension graft to connect the medial crura with the anterior septum, or strengthening the medial crura with an extended columellar strut. The choice of graft depends on each patient's specific anatomic deficiencies and surgical goals.

The patient who has a hanging columella and prominent caudal septum that would otherwise require trimming will benefit from a medial crural setback on the midline caudal septum. To perform the setback, bilateral mucoperichondrial flaps are raised after dissecting between the medial crura to expose the septum (**Fig. 16**A). Then the medial crura are sutured to the extra length of the caudal septum. Rather than trimming the excessive caudal septum, it is left in place to support the medial crura, which are fixed using a 4-0 plain catgut suture on a straight septal needle (**Fig. 16**B). This method, described by Kridel and colleagues,[10] can be used instead of placing a columellar strut.[4] Before suturing, the caudal septum must be in the midline; otherwise, the tip will be deviated. After initial fixation, careful assessment of tip projection, nasolabial angle, alar-columellar relationship, and tip rotation is critical to avoid deformity. The fixation suture between the caudal septum and medial crus should be placed through the crus's cephalic margin to avoid retraction of the columella. When all parameters have been set appropriately, the position is stabilized with a 5-0 clear nylon suture, which is placed from the internal surface of the intermediate crura along its cephalic margin to the caudal septum. After this suture is placed, the domes and medial crura should be symmetric. This maneuver is only appropriate in patients who have a redundancy of caudal septal length that would otherwise require trimming. Ideal candidates for this technique include patients who have a hanging columella because of a long caudal septum (**Fig. 17**) and patients who have a short upper lip, because fixation of the medial crura to the caudal septum will usually lengthen the upper lip.

For the patient who has a caudal septum that is short or of appropriate length, base stabilization is best accomplished using a caudal extension graft. The graft creates a stable fixation point for medial crura fixation, and the foreshortened septum can be appropriately lengthened simultaneously (**Fig. 18**).[4,11] The choice of grafting material to create a caudal extension graft should be a relatively straight segment of cartilage, which is secured to the existing caudal septum end-to-end or in an overlapping position (**Fig. 19**).[11] Inherent deviations in the caudal septum or the extension graft are used to one's advantage to position the tip structure in the midline. If the caudal septum has a slight curve to the left, the graft would be placed to the right. Similarly, if the graft and caudal septum both have a slight curvature, the two cartilages can be sutured together with their concave surfaces opposing each other to create a straighter layered unit. If overlapping the caudal extension graft creates unavoidable deformity regardless of its orientation, then this graft can be placed end to end with the septum and stabilized with thin splinting cartilage grafts placed on both sides of the junction to ensure that the graft is midline. Analogous to the functions of the splinting grafts, extralong extended spreader grafts can be placed such that their most distal ends project beyond the caudal septum to overlie and fix the caudal extension graft placed end to end.[7]

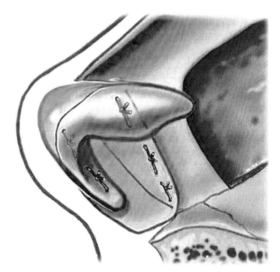

**Fig. 18.** The caudal extension graft can be placed end-to-end or overlap the existing caudal septum and is sutured with at least two 5-0 clear nylon sutures. This graft is rectangular in shape to provide support with little change in rotation or nasal length. The caudal margin of this graft must be in the midline; otherwise, the tip may deviate or the airway may be obstructed. A 4-0 plain catgut suture and 5-0 clear nylon suture are used to fix the medial crura to the caudal extension graft.

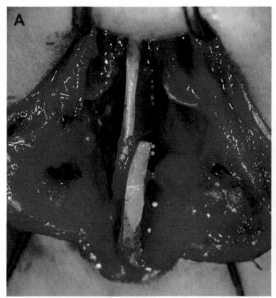

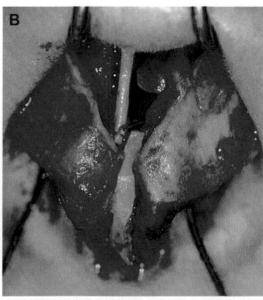

**Fig. 19.** Caudal extension graft. (*A*) The caudal extension graft is overlapping the existing caudal septum. Care is taken to make sure the caudal margin of the extension graft is in the midline and that the cephalic margin is not blocking the airway. The caudal septum was slightly deviated to the patient's right in this case, so the caudal extension graft was overlapped on the left. The extension graft has a slight curvature to bring the caudal margin back to the midline. (*B*) The medial crura are sutured to the caudal margin of the extension graft with multiple 5-0 clear nylon sutures. Note the midline tip structure.

The caudal extension graft has a great deal of versatility to modify tip position. Depending on the shape and orientation of the caudal extension graft, it can alter the nasolabial angle, tip rotation, nasal length, and columella–ala relationship. For the ptotic nasal tip with an acute nasolabial angle, the caudal extension graft is crafted with a longer inferior margin to achieve tip rotation (**Fig. 20**). The longer inferior extension will blunt the acute nasolabial angle and stabilize the base of the nose (**Fig. 21**). For an overrotated nose with a short dorsal length, the extension graft is shaped with a longer superior margin to counter rotate the nasal tip and lengthen the nose by pushing the tip down (**Fig. 22**). Once the graft is in position, the medial crura can then be sutured to the caudal margin of the caudal extension graft with 5-0 clear nylon sutures to stabilize the base of the nose, set tip position, and create an appropriate columella–ala relationship. The nylon sutures are placed through the internal surface of the intermediate crura and then fixed to the caudal extension graft. Symmetry of these sutures is critical to avoid tip deformity and establish dome symmetry. For maximum support, additional fixation can secure the caudal extension graft to the nasal spine periosteum inferiorly, and either paired splinting grafts or extended spreader grafts can provide additional lateral support superiorly. Any overlapping grafts along the cephalic margin can create extra bulk

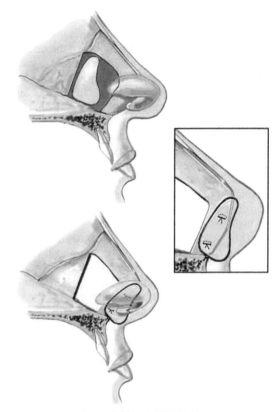

**Fig. 20.** A caudal extension graft used for correction of the ptotic nasal tip with acute nasolabial angle. A contoured septal cartilage graft that is longer along the inferior margin is used to augment the nasolabial angle and rotate the nasal tip. This graft can be fixed to the periosteum around the nasal spine to stabilize the graft further.

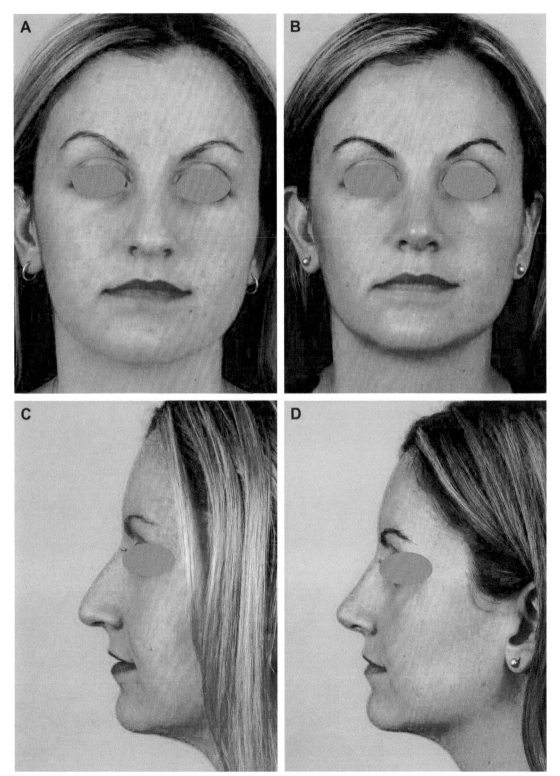

Fig. 21. This patient had a modest retraction of her nasolabial angle with weakness in her nasal base. She under-went placement of a caudal extension graft to augment her nasolabial angle. The graft was longer along its in-ferior margin. Dome sutures were used after placing lateral crural strut grafts to flatten the lateral crura. A bruised cartilage graft was placed horizontally over the domes to provide additional tip definition. *A, C, E,* and *G* are preoperative views; *B, D, F* and *H* are 1-year postoperative views.

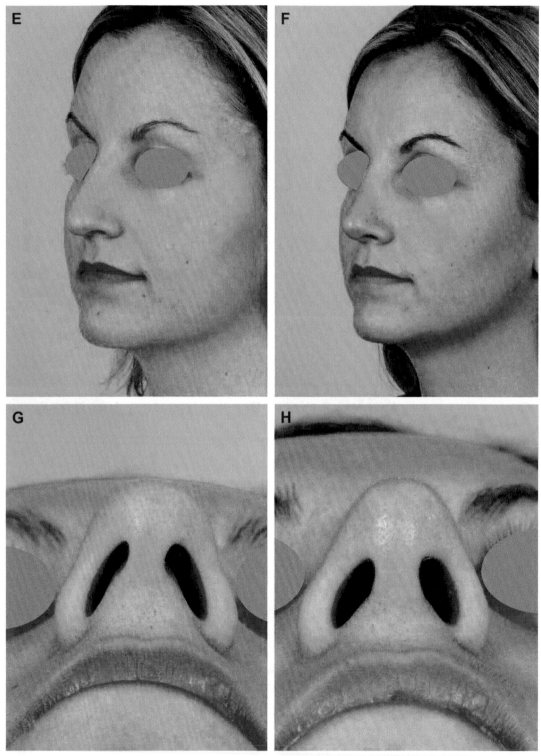

**Fig. 21.** (*continued*).

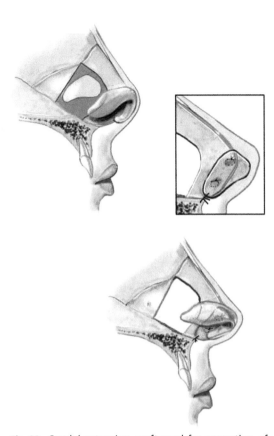

Fig. 22. Caudal extension graft used for correction of the foreshortened nose. This graft is longer along its superior border to counter rotate the tip and lengthen the nose. The graft can be further stabilized using bilateral extended spreader grafts.

that may obstruct the airway and should thus be trimmed or beveled to maximize the nasal airway space. One can easily create a deformity or airway obstruction if these grafts are not placed properly; therefore, use of the caudal extension graft requires accurate diagnosis of contour defects before correctly placing the graft to establish a natural tip position. Patients undergoing placement of caudal extension grafts should be warned during preoperative consultation that their noses will be stiffer and have less tip recoil.

In patients in whom the base of the nose is severely deficient or major augmentation of the premaxilla is needed, the surgeon can use an extended columellar strut with or without a premaxillary graft. When the extended columellar strut is placed without a premaxillary graft for modest augmentation of the premaxilla, it is placed in a pocket between the medial crura and fixed directly to the nasal spine by way of three

possible techniques. First, it can be sutured to thin splinting grafts placed bilaterally, which are, in turn, sutured to the nasal spine through a predrilled hole using a 16-gauge needle (**Fig. 23**). Alternatively, the graft can be carved with a flare at the base of the strut and a notch cut in the posterior surface of the graft to sit over the nasal spine and allow the caudal septum to integrate with the graft (**Fig. 24**).[4,12] In either technique, the bases of the grafts are fixed with two 4-0 polydioxanone (PDS) sutures applied through the nasal spine. The third and final technique secures the strut reliably and is adjustable for a paramedian-situated nasal spine. In this technique, a notch is created in the bony maxilla using a 5-mm osteotome. The notch is placed either through the nasal spine or just lateral to it, where the new center of the nasal base should be. The extended columellar strut is then slotted into the notch and fixed with two 4-0 PDS sutures tied directly to the bone through a similarly predrilled hole (**Fig. 25**). The amount of premaxilla augmentation is directly proportional to the degree of caudal extension of the extended columella

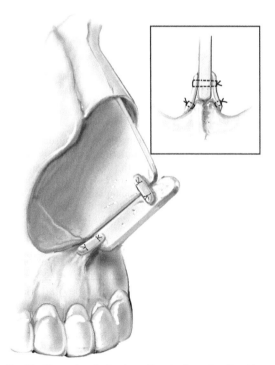

Fig. 23. The extended columellar strut can be fixed to the nasal spine region by using paired splinting grafts on both sides of the nasal spine to stabilize the graft in the midline. As seen in the inset, the splinting grafts are secured by suturing through predrilled holes in the bony spine.

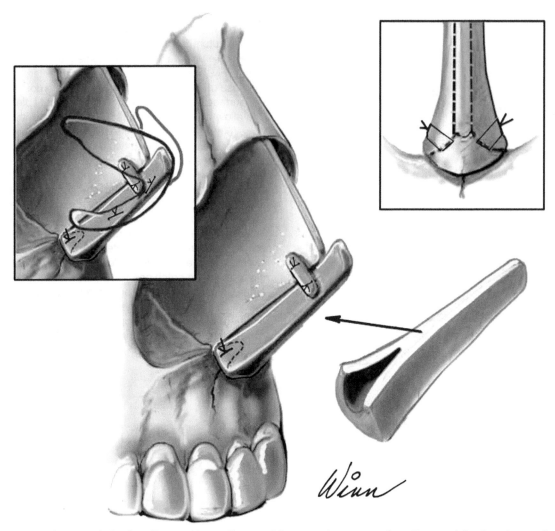

**Fig. 24.** The extended columellar strut is usually carved from autologous costal cartilage and fixed to the nasal spine periosteum or to a notch in a premaxillary graft. To aid in fixation, a notch can be created at the base of the strut to integrate with the nasal spine and premaxilla. Splinting grafts can be sandwiched on both sides of the graft to stabilize the graft superiorly. In the left inset, note how the lower lateral cartilages are suture fixated to the extended columellar strut.

graft that extends to the nasal spine. The nasal length and columella–ala relationship are also controlled by the caudal extension of the graft. Rotation of the tip can be controlled precisely by altering the angle of the graft before securing the anterior projection to extended spreader grafts from above. Tip projection is determined by graft length, and columellar width on base view is directly proportional to graft thickness. The extended columella graft is a powerful technique that also enables the surgeon to correct deviations of the nasal base from midline. When the nasal spine does not align with a vertical line dropped down from the nasion, the extended columellar graft can be placed left or right of the nasal spine to correct for this deviation. The combination of an extended columella graft and a premaxillary graft is useful to maximize augmentation of the premaxilla. The premaxillary graft is placed, depending on its size, either through the medial intercrural pocket or through a separate sublabial incision. It is sutured directly to the nasal spine with suture either through the periosteum or a predrilled hole. A notch carved on the anterior surface of the premaxillary graft supports the extended columellar graft (**Fig. 26**). Regardless of the

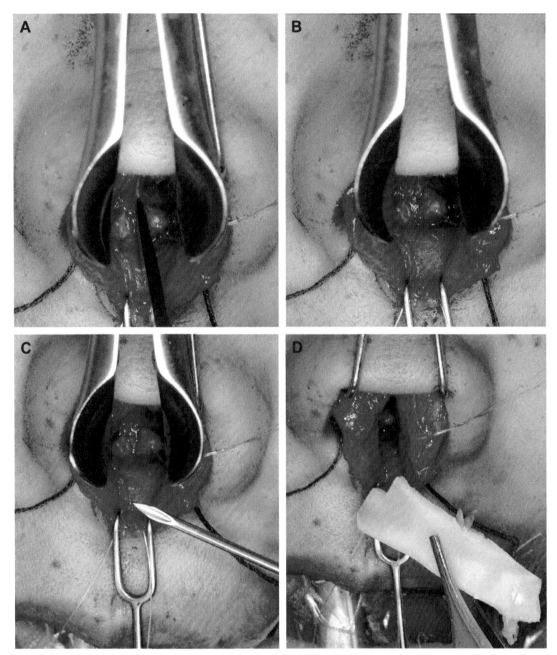

Fig. 25. The extended columellar strut can also be fixed to the nasal spine by creating a notch in the nasal spine and setting the graft inside the notch. (A) The nasal spine is notched with a 5-mm osteotome. (B) The notch is made at the center of the nasal spine so each splayed half of bony spine serves as a splint for the graft. (C) A 16-gauge needle is used to drill a hole through the nasal spine posterior to the notch. (D) The extended columellar strut is carved with a corner cut out to create a groove. This groove secures the graft, once placed in the notch, to prevent anterior or posterior movement of the graft.

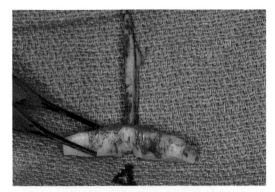

**Fig. 26.** For maximal premaxillary augmentation, the extended columellar strut can be integrated into a notch in a premaxillary graft placed into a pocket over the premaxilla.

specific type of extended columellar strut used, all can significantly alter tip position and projection. These patients should be told that their nasal tip will be rigid and stiff postoperatively.

### Controlling Nasal Tip Contour

After adequate base stabilization, the nasal tip can be contoured reliably. Specific techniques are aimed at manipulating the underlying anatomic supporting structures to create the desired external contour. Application of good techniques for the wrong diagnosis will only frustrate the surgeon and patient alike. Therefore, the following techniques are grouped by indication and, when appropriate, common errors are presented to reinforce the correct application.

Patients who present with a nasal tip that is broad, bulbous, or poorly defined commonly request a narrower tip. The surgeon must assess the horizontal and vertical contributions to the tip bulbosity. Management of the nasal tip typically requires manipulating the lower lateral cartilages in both the horizontal (dome to dome) and vertical (caudal margin to cephalic margin) dimensions. The surgeon must also determine whether the lateral crura are oriented properly. Thus, techniques will vary to specifically address horizontal versus vertical excess and will vary to correct lateral crural malpositioning, if present. Considering first the scenario with normal orientation of the lateral crura but too much vertical height (excess cartilage width from caudal to cephalic margins), one will find supratip fullness noted on lateral view. To correct this, a conservative cephalic trim of the lateral

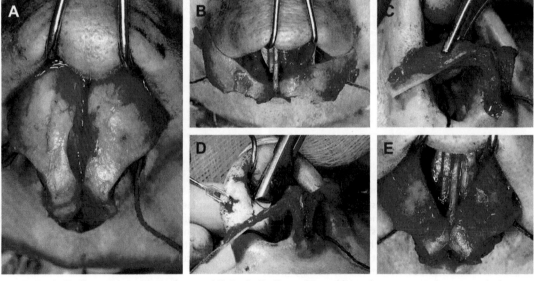

**Fig. 27.** Cephalically positioned lateral crura. (*A*) Cephalically positioned lateral crura create excess vertical supratip fullness. Before manipulation, the caudal margin of the lateral crura lies below the cephalic margin. (*B*) The lateral crura are dissected from the underlying vestibular skin. (*C*) Lateral crural strut grafts are sutured to the undersurface of the lateral crura with 5-0 clear nylon sutures. (*D*) A more caudally positioned pocket is created to accommodate the lateral crus. (*E*) After lateral crural strut grafts are sutured to the undersurface of the lateral crura, the lateral crura are repositioned into the new, caudally positioned pockets to correct the cephalic positioning. After graft placement and repositioning, the lateral crura are now oriented close to 45° off midline instead of the preoperative cephalic orientation.

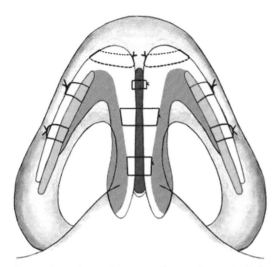

**Fig. 28.** Lateral crural strut grafts are shown in light blue. These cartilage grafts are sutured to the undersurface of the lateral crura to flatten the crura and eliminate the bulbous contour of the nasal tip. After the lateral crural strut grafts are placed, dome sutures can be positioned to narrow the domes and decrease the dome angle. Note how the 5-0 clear nylon sutures are oriented with the knots above the lateral crura. The dark blue structure between the medial crura represents a strut or caudal extension graft.

crura will decrease vertical height and supratip fullness; however, cephalic trim of the lateral crura is not the primary method used to decrease supratip fullness. It may also be necessary to trim the anterior septal angle if it approaches the level of the domes. For the patient who has normal orientation of the lateral crura and a component of horizontal

excess, the excessive interdomal distance creates a wide tip on frontal and base views. In this case, dome sutures are also an effective means of decreasing supratip fullness. Generally, it is usually appropriate to narrow the nasal tip by performing a conservative cephalic trim, leaving 8 to 10 mm of lateral crus laterally and approximately 5 to 7 mm medially at the domes. When the lower lateral cartilage width at the dome is narrow, it is best not to perform medial cartilage excision near the domes or this will weaken them. The ideal location for a cephalic trim is the medial two thirds of the lateral crura. Thinning the lateral third of the lateral crus leads to supra-alar pinching and lateral wall collapse with nasal obstruction, which are common findings in patients who have undergone rhinoplasty and tend to worsen significantly over time. In fact, the senior author routinely places alar batten grafts in a pocket just medial to the supra-alar crease as a prophylactic maneuver to prevent collapse of the lateral wall.[13]

Patients who have malpositioning of the lateral crura require a completely different approach, which includes reorienting the lateral crura. Patients commonly have cephalically oriented lateral crura instead of the more normal oblique orientation ranging from 35° to 45° off midline. The combination of bulbous and cephalically orientated lateral crura typically create a "parentheses" appearance on frontal view.[1] In these patients, it is recommended to perform a conservative cephalic trim and dissect the lateral crura from the vestibular skin, suture lateral crural strut grafts to the undersurfaces of the lateral crura, and then reposition the lateral crura into caudally positioned pockets (**Fig. 27**).[14] The lateral crural strut grafts

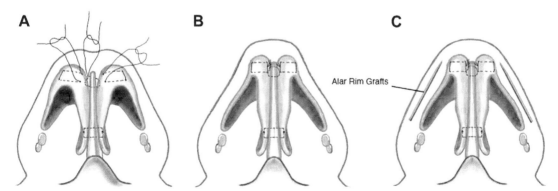

**Fig. 29.** (A) Placement of two separate 5-0 clear nylon dome sutures will narrow the dome angle. Then, a 5-0 clear nylon interdomal suture sets the width between the domes. (B) Note some pinching at the junction between the tip lobule and alar lobule, which will require placement of alar rim grafts to reposition the alar margin and avoid a visible transition from tip lobule to alar lobule. (C) Note how the alar rim grafts create a triangular shape to the nasal base.

act to flatten the bulbous lateral crura and create a more favorable tip contour. Repositioning the lateral crura places supportive cartilage along the sidewall of the nose to prevent lateral wall collapse. This maneuver also acts to create a more favorable position of the caudal margin of the lateral crura relative to the cephalic margin (see **Fig. 8**). If the cephalically positioned lateral crura are flat and do not contribute to tip bulbosity or middle vault width, they can be left in position using alar batten grafts to support the lateral nasal wall.

Overall tip shape extends well beyond the tip lobule. Dome-binding sutures are a good way to decrease the horizontal contribution of the bulbous nasal tip contour in the primary rhinoplasty patient. The dome sutures act to variably narrow the dome angle, depending on the stiffness of the lateral crura and on how tightly the sutures are tied. Dome sutures have lateral effects, too, which ultimately enable the surgeon to contour the transition between the tip lobule and lateral alae. The objective of placing dome sutures is to create flat lateral crura; however, in most cases, some degree of concavity will be noted.[3] In patients who have soft cartilages, the dome sutures will tend to pinch and deform the dome and leave convexity between the dome and the lateral aspect of the lateral crus. If the lateral crura do not flatten properly but instead deform or buckle with placement of the suture, then a lateral crural strut graft sutured to the undersurface of the lateral crus can be used (**Fig. 28**).[14] The lateral crural strut grafts are thin, but stiff, pieces of cartilage designed to counteract any lateral buckling or convexity of the lateral crus seen after placement of the dome sutures. When combined with dome sutures, these grafts will flatten the lateral crura, resulting in a refined nasal tip with good transition from tip lobule to both alae.

Using two separate interrupted dome sutures is usually preferred over a single transdomal suture, to prevent pinching the domes together. The sutures are placed in a horizontal mattress fashion, tying the knots medially between the domes (**Fig. 29**). Symmetric placement along the axis of the anatomic dome will slightly rotate the nasal tip lobule. By using two separate dome sutures, the normal divergence of the intermediate crura can be preserved. Surgeons frequently err by trying to narrow the tip further by bringing the domes too close together. Unfortunately, this maneuver will tend to obliterate the normal columellar-lobular angle, excessively narrow the tip, and create a vertical orientation instead of the normal horizontal orientation of the nasal tip highlight. Preservation of the divergence between the intermediate crura

keeps the desirable columellar-lobular angle or double break (see **Fig. 15**).[1] A separate interdomal suture of 5-0 clear nylon placed from the internal surface of both intermediate crura sets the width between the domes (see **Fig. 28**). This suture should not be tied too tightly; otherwise, the domes will be too close together, creating abnormal anatomy. By using a transdomal suture (a single dome suture that pinches both domes together) or other tip-narrowing methods that unify the domes, the divergence between the intermediate crura may be eliminated and the columellar-lobular angle can be mistakenly blunted.

After placing the dome sutures, the support and contour of the alar margins can be reconstituted to recreate the elevated ridge along the alar margin that transitions from tip to alar lobule. Recall that descent of the lateral crus below the cephalic margin (see **Fig. 9**) and lateral crural concavity (see **Fig. 29**B) are two deformities that disrupt this lateral alar contour, and completely reversing them is not always possible. An alternative method of repositioning the alar margin to create favorable tip contour is to place alar rim grafts into pockets along the caudal margin of the marginal incision (**Fig. 30**).[4,15] The alar rim grafts recreate the elevated ridge between the tip and alar lobule and fill

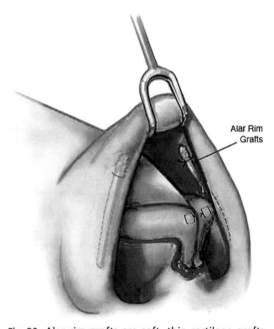

Alar Rim
Grafts

**Fig. 30.** Alar rim grafts are soft, thin cartilage grafts placed into a pocket along the caudal margin of the marginal incision. Note how the medial margins of the grafts are crushed to make them soft after they are sutured to the surrounding soft tissue. The sutures are placed around the graft to avoid fracture.

the void created by any concavity of the lateral crura or descent of the caudal margin of the lateral crura. Alar rim grafts typically are thin, soft cartilage grafts that measure approximately 12- to 15-mm long and 2- to 3-mm wide (**Fig. 31**). A converse scissors is used to create a pocket along the caudal margin of the marginal incision. Special care is taken not to puncture the skin of the alar lobule by staying close to the vestibular skin. Then, the alar rim graft is placed into the pocket and sutured to surrounding soft tissue with a 6-0 Monocryl (Ethicon Inc., Somerville, New Jersey) suture by tying around the graft to avoid fracturing the cartilage. Before closure, the medial margin of the alar rim graft is gently crushed with Brown-Adson forceps to reduce the risk for visibility or palpability of the graft. If the alar rim grafts are too long or are not

crushed medially, a risk is presented for leaving a visible irregularity in the nasal tip postoperatively. The combination of conservative cephalic trim, dome-binding sutures, and alar rim grafts can correct a bulbous tip effectively and create the desired contour of the nasal tip (**Fig. 32**).

The preoperative state of some patients' lower lateral cartilages may show the caudal margin below the cephalic margin. Many of these patients possess a favorable tip contour owing to the soft tissue contributions along the alar lobule and do not need alar rim grafts. Patients who have thicker skin (eg, Asian and other nonwhite patients) may have adequate support of the alar lobule from the thick skin and soft tissues. Alar rim grafts are used in patients who have a narrow (pinched), poorly balanced nasal tip. In these patients, alar

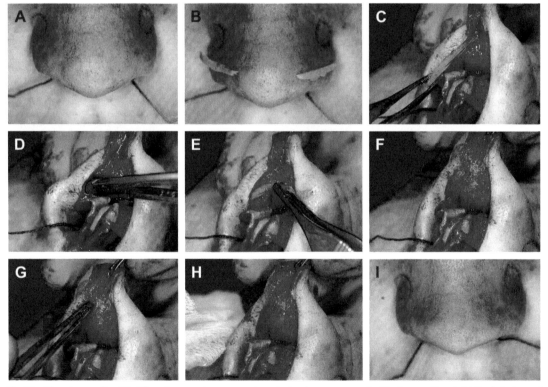

**Fig. 31.** Alar rim grafts. (*A*) After dome sutures are placed, shadows are created between the right tip lobule and the alar lobule. The tip contour is unfavorable. (*B*) Alar rim grafts are placed about 3 mm caudally to the alar margin. (*C*) The grafts are thin and measure around 12 to 15 mm in length. (*D*) Converse scissors are used to make a narrow pocket along the caudal margin of the marginal incision. The pocket extends laterally and is made closer to the internal vestibular skin so that the graft is not visible postoperatively. (*E*) The thin strip of cartilage is placed into the pocket. (*F*) Suture fixation with 6-0 Monocryl passed through soft tissue and around the graft. (*G*) Brown-Adson forceps are used to crush the medial margin of the graft. (*H*) Note how the medial margin of the graft is soft, so it will not be visible in the tip. (*I*) After alar rim grafts are placed, deeper shadows are created in the supra-alar region, and the shadow between the tip lobule and alar lobule is eliminated. A prominence, or ridge, extends from the tip to the alar lobule that aids in defining the supra-alar shadows. These changes represent the elevation of the alar lobule with placement of the alar rim grafts.

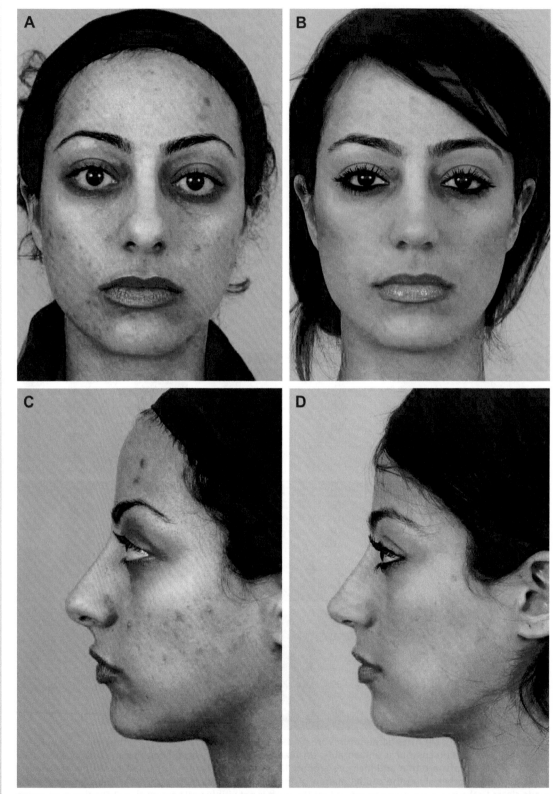

**Fig. 32.** Patient who had a bulbous nasal tip treated with conservative cephalic trim, lateral crural strut grafts, dome sutures, and bilateral alar rim grafts. The caudal septum was long, but it was not trimmed. Instead, the medial crura were sutured to the caudal septum to stabilize the base of the nose. The medial crura were sutured to the caudal septum in a slightly deprojected position. A, C, E, and G are preoperative views; B, D, F, and H are 1-year postoperative views. (*From* Toriumi DM. New concepts in nasal tip contouring. Arch Facial Plast Surg 2006;8:156–185; with permission. Copyright © 2006, American Medical Association. All rights reserved.)

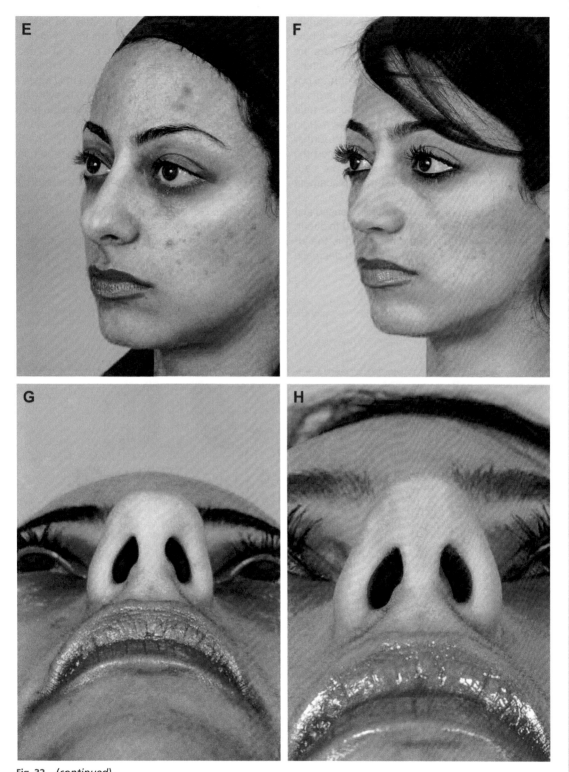

**Fig. 32.** (continued).

rim grafts will support and elevate the alar margin, creating a good transition from tip to alar lobule with a horizontal tip highlight. Alar rim grafts are usually not necessary in patients who have lateral crura that extend caudally beyond the normal position or in patients in whom the caudal margin of the lateral crura is appropriately positioned near the same horizontal plane as the cephalic margin (see **Figs. 7, 8**). Lateral crura that extend further caudally than normal can be identified when the marginal incision must be positioned more caudally than normal, leaving little room for placement of an alar rim graft.

After placement of alar rim grafts, increased alar flare and enlargement of the nostrils tend to occur. A consequence of using alar rim grafts is the increased need for alar base reduction to decrease the alar flare and nostril size. Usually, an internal alar base reduction, taking a triangle of skin at the junction between the ala and nostril sill, is necessary to correct this problem. Incisions made in this area of the nose can create unsightly scars if not executed properly. In an effort to evert the skin edge, one can create a subtle favorable bevel with the excision (**Fig. 33**). This bevel should be symmetric and angle no greater than 10° to 15° from the perpendicular. An excessive or improper bevel will result in an unsightly scar. A 6-0 PDS suture is used to approximate the subcutaneous tissues. Multiple 7-0 vertical mattress nylon sutures are used to close the beveled skin edge to ensure precise alignment. Unlike the midcolumellar sutures, which are removed 1 week after surgery, the alar-base sutures remain 2 weeks

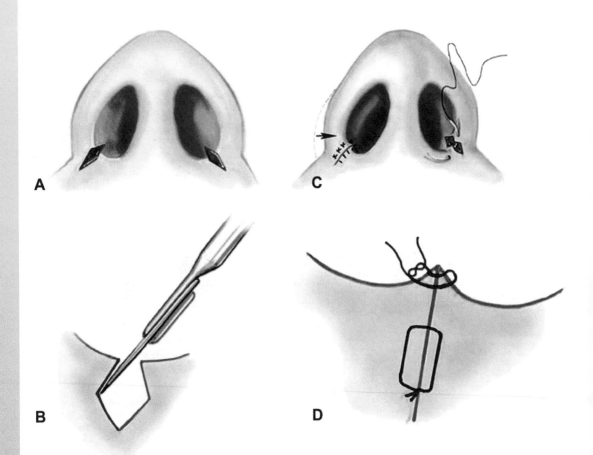

**Fig. 33.** Alar base reduction after placement of alar rim grafts. (A) Small, triangular, wedged segments of skin are excised near the junction between the nostril and nostril sill. The excision will make the nostril smaller and decrease flare of the alar margin created by placement of the alar rim grafts. (B) The excision is executed with a slight favorable bevel of the skin excision to promote eversion of the skin edges with closure. (C) 5-0 PDS subcutaneous suture is placed, followed by skin closure with 7-0 nylon vertical mattress sutures. (D) Appropriate skin edge eversion is illustrated by the cross-section schematic of the deep and superficial sutures.

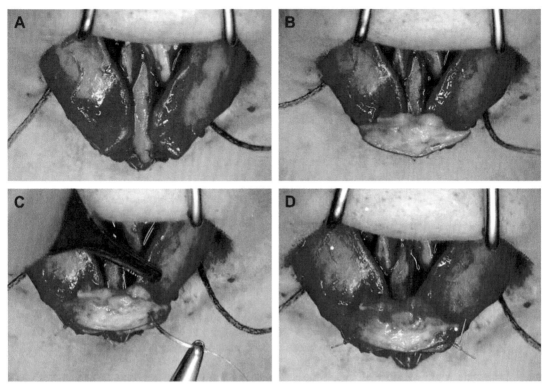

**Fig. 34.** Soft cartilage (cephalic trim of lateral crus) can be sutured across the domes to provide additional projection and definition. (*A*) Domes after placement of separate dome sutures and interdomal suture to set interdomal distance. Note that the normal divergence between the intermediate crura is preserved. (*B*) Orientation of soft cartilage graft (cephalic trim of lateral crus) across domes (horizontally oriented). The graft sits along the caudal margin of the domes and extends lateral to the domes. (*C*) 6-0 Monocryl sutures are used to fix the graft. (*D*) Note how the graft is relatively flat, thus avoiding postoperative visibility.

postoperatively to resist the extra skin tension at this incision. If not performed precisely, base reductions present a high risk for visible scars and deformities, such as small or asymmetric nostrils, notched nostril sill, or altered alar insertions. This maneuver is extremely technique sensitive and adds at least 40 more minutes to the procedure time; therefore, it should not be attempted if the surgeon is not able to take the additional time necessary to execute these maneuvers properly.

Additional fine tuning to the tip projection and contour definition are frequently enhanced with soft, gently crushed cartilage grafts, which can be sutured horizontally across both domes with 6-0 Monocryl suture. The graft should be sutured to the caudal margin of the domes to ensure that the caudal margin of the dome structure is raised above the cephalic margin, and it should extend laterally just beyond the domes to act as camouflage.

These grafts can provide further definition to the horizontal tip highlight, increase projection to refine tip narrowing, and soften the transition from dome to alar lobule laterally. The soft cartilage excised during the cephalic trim of the lateral crura is ideal for this graft because it contains soft tissue, which contains the crushed cartilage fragments and improves its fixation to the domes (**Fig. 34**). The importance of gently crushing the cartilage with Brown-Adson forceps or a block-type morcellizer reduces the risk for graft visibility postoperatively. In patients who have very thin skin, such grafts should be avoided because graft visibility is likely.

Routine use of shield tip grafts to increase tip projection in primary rhinoplasty is unnecessary when the surgeon can work with the patient's existing domes. Tip projection can be controlled in most primary rhinoplasty patients by grafting and stabilizing the base (columellar strut graft, fixing

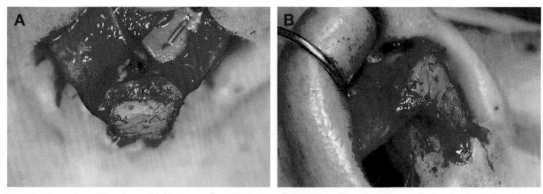

**Fig. 35.** The sutured-in-place shield tip graft. (*A*) The graft is camouflaged with a soft, bruised cartilage graft sutured behind the leading edge of the graft. (*B*) Note how the soft graft extends laterally to the margins of the tip graft to help with the transitions to the existing lateral crura.

medial crura to caudal septum, caudal extension graft, or extended columellar strut graft) followed by placement of dome sutures and soft cartilage grafts positioned over the domes to project and further refine the tip.[4,11–13] In some patients needing tip projection, the lower lateral cartilages are very weak or diminutive and will not provide adequate projection with suturing methods alone. In such patients, sutured-in-place shield grafts can be used to help project and define the tip.[8] Shield grafts are used mainly in secondary rhinoplasty, in augmentation rhinoplasty, or in primary rhinoplasty patients who have an underprojected tip with thick skin and a deficient tip lobule. If one does use a shield tip graft, it must be properly carved and camouflaged to avoid visibility of the graft, because the skin tends to thin and contract over time.[4,12,13] Any shield graft that projects above the existing domes is at risk for becoming visible, regardless of skin thickness. The sutured-in-place shield graft is best camouflaged using bruised or gently crushed cartilage placed around the leading edge of the graft (**Fig. 35**). The softened cartilage will create a smooth transition from shield tip graft to the lateral crura and will camouflage the graft. If the shield tip graft projects more than 3 mm above the existing domes, crushed cartilage alone is not sufficient, and lateral crural grafts are typically added to create a smooth transition from the lateral margin of the shield tip graft to the existing lateral crura (**Fig. 36**). Pressure of the skin envelope on a shield tip graft will tend to rotate the graft cephalically, causing a blunted infratip lobule. The lateral crural grafts will support the graft from behind and prevent the shield graft from tilting cephalically, which is particularly important when the shield tip graft is projected into a thick, tight skin envelope (**Fig. 37**). The lateral crural grafts are oriented at a 45° angle from midline and taper back onto the lateral crura, where

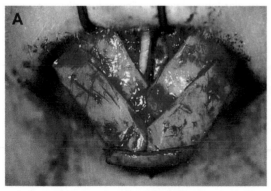
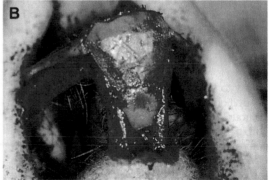

**Fig. 36.** Shield tip grafts that project over 3 mm above the existing domes are stabilized with lateral crural grafts. (*A*) These grafts are oriented obliquely off the posterior surface of the tip graft and then sutured to the lateral crura. (*B*) The lateral crural grafts typically overlap the lateral crura by at least 5 mm.

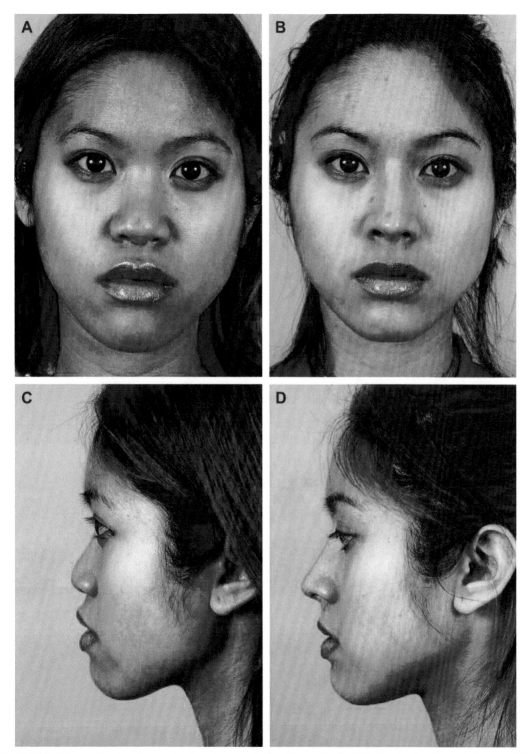

**Fig. 37.** This Asian patient underwent prior placement of a silicone implant that extruded through her nasal tip and left a scar. Reconstruction required use of a costal cartilage extended columellar strut fixed to the nasal spine periosteum. A costal cartilage dorsal graft was also used. A shield tip graft with lateral crural grafts was used to contour the nasal tip. The tip graft was covered with a layer of perichondrium from costal cartilage. *A, C, E,* and *G* are preoperative views; *B, D, F,* and *H* are 2-year postoperative views. Note the change in the nasolabial angle with the extended columellar strut. The shield graft is supported from behind with the lateral crural grafts to prevent cephalic rotation and provide improved nasal tip definition with a horizontal tip orientation. (*From* Toriumi DM. New concepts in nasal tip contouring. Arch Facial Plast Surg 2006;8:156–185; with permission. Copyright © 2006, American Medical Association. All rights reserved.)

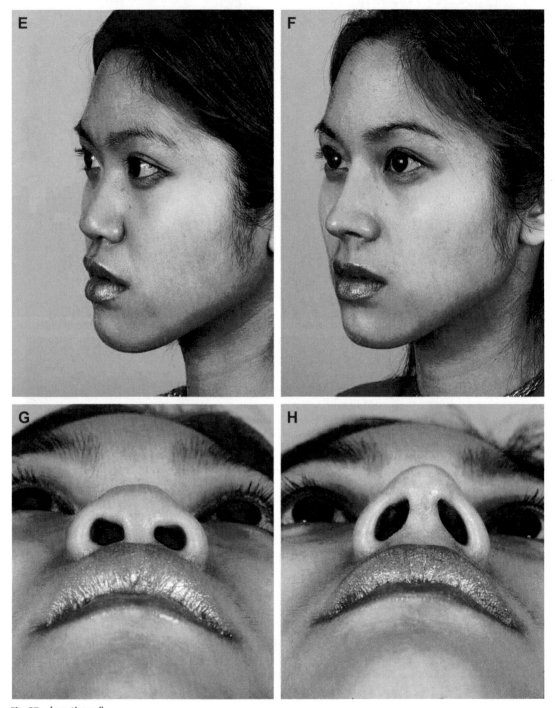

**Fig. 37.** (*continued*).

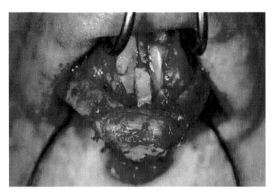

**Fig. 38.** Perichondrium is sutured over the tip graft and lateral crural grafts to help ensure a smooth contour and to help camouflage the tip graft.

they are sutured in place with 6-0 Monocryl suture. Lateral crural grafts should not be confused with lateral crural strut grafts, which are sutured to the undersurface of the lateral crura adjacent to the vestibular skin. A sheet of gently crushed cartilage can be placed over the shield graft and lateral crural graft construction to camouflage the grafts further. If available, perichondrium harvested from either conchal bowl or costal cartilage, instead of gently crushed cartilage, can be placed over the entire shield tip graft reconstruction to provide additional camouflage (**Fig. 38**).[13] Alar rim grafts are then placed along the caudal aspect of the marginal incisions to create a transition off the lateral margin of the shield tip graft and create the appropriate shadows and highlights of the nasal tip. In some cases, it is necessary to suture the medial margin of the alar rim graft to the lateral margin of the shield graft. This procedure will help camouflage the lateral margin of the shield graft. With the combination of nasal base support, shield graft with lateral crural grafts and alar rim grafts, and appropriate camouflage, nearly complete tip reconstructions can be executed, creating natural-appearing tip contours in secondary and augmentation rhinoplasty (**Fig. 39**).[16] Even for complex nasal tip reconstructions, creating favorable shadows with a horizontally oriented tip highlight is the ultimate goal.

## SUMMARY

Nasal tip contouring is a complex endeavor that requires proper execution of several complimentary techniques. Success is achieved not by mastering the techniques alone, but rather, by simultaneously analyzing existing contour deformities, the causative structural deficiencies or anomalies, and the exterior effects that graft insertion and cartilage manipulation yield. The surgeon's ability to

achieve his/her envisioned external nasal tip shape is only possible after minimizing all the potential risks for negative outcomes that present with each technical maneuver. One must be acutely aware of the numerous undesirable consequences of wound contracture, graft show, cartilage bending or warping, asymmetries, or scarring, just to name a few. Many deformities noted after rhinoplasty are created by using techniques incorrectly or by neglecting to anticipate postoperative changes like skin thinning or scar contracture.

The use of nasal tip narrowing techniques that tend to pinch the domes and create an abnormal shadow between the tip lobule and alar lobule should be avoided. For a more natural appearance to the nasal tip, the goal should be to create a horizontally oriented tip highlight that transitions smoothly from tip lobule to alar lobule. This result is best accomplished by stabilizing the base of the nose, conservatively suturing the tip, applying appropriate grafting techniques, and placing alar rim grafts. Pearls to remember that will lead to increased success in contouring the nasal tip include

Strategic placement of highlights and shadows creates a more natural-appearing tip.

A clear understanding of the three-dimensional topography of the ideal tip frees the surgeon from dwelling on specific maneuvers to focus on creating the intended shape.

Careful attention to detail will lengthen the duration of surgery and requires patience and persistence.

A commitment to this method of surgery will make predetermined aesthetic goals more obtainable and predictable while avoiding the stigma of the operated-looking nose.

88

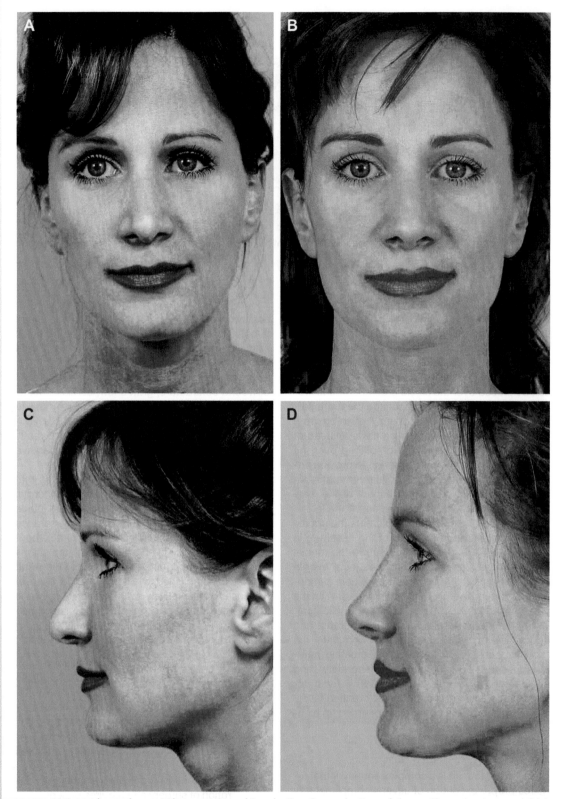

**Fig. 39.** Patient who underwent three previous rhinoplasties. Overreduction of the cartilage structure and thick skin resulted in a constricted ball appearance to the nasal tip and pollybeak deformity. Correction required a tip graft with lateral crural grafts. A cartilage dorsal graft was used to increase dorsal height. The nose was made larger on the lateral view to expand the thick skin and create a more defined frontal view. Note the horizontally oriented nasal tip highlight on the postoperative frontal view. *A, C, E,* and *G* are preoperative views; *B, D, F,* and *H* are 2-year postoperative views. (*From* Toriumi DM. New concepts in nasal tip contouring. Arch Facial Plast Surg 2006;8:156–185; with permission. Copyright © 2006, American Medical Association. All rights reserved.)

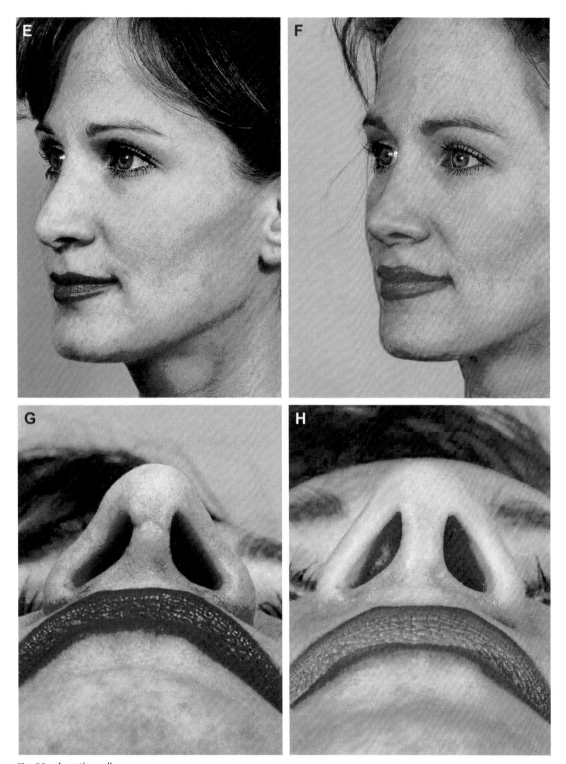

**Fig. 39.** *(continued).*

## REFERENCES

1. Sheen JH, Sheen AP. Aesthetic rhinoplasty. 2nd edition. St Louis (Mo): CV Mosby; 1987.
2. Tardy ME. Rhinoplasty: the art and the science. Philadelphia: WB Saunders Co; 1996.
3. Daniel RK. The nasal tip: anatomy and aesthetics. Plast Reconstr Surg 1992;89:216–24.
4. Toriumi DM. Structure approach in rhinoplasty. Facial Plast Surg Clin North Am 2005;13:93–113.
5. Gunter JP, Rohrich RJ, Friedman RM. Classification and correction of alarcolumellar discrepancies in rhinoplasty. Plast Reconstr Surg 1996;97:643–8.
6. Guyuron B, DeLuca L, Lash R. Supratip deformity: a closer look. Plast Reconstr Surg 2000;105:1140–51.
7. Ha RY, Byrd HS. Septal extension grafts revisited: 6-year experience in controlling nasal tip projection and shape. Plast Reconstr Surg 2003;112:1929–35.
8. Johnson CMJ, Toriumi DM. Open structure rhinoplasty. Philadelphia: WB Saunders Co; 1989.
9. Johnson CMJ, Godin MS. The tension nose: open structure rhinoplasty approach. Plast Reconstr Surg 1995;95:43–5.
10. Kridel RWH, Scott BA, Foda HMT. The tongue-in-groove technique in septorhinoplasty: a 10-year experience. Arch Facial Plast Surg. 1999;1:246–56.
11. Toriumi DM. Caudal septal extension graft for correction of the retracted columella. Op Tech Otolaryngol Head Neck Surg. 1995;6:311–8.
12. Toriumi DM. Structure concept in nasal tip surgery. Op Tech Plast Reconstr Surg. 2000;7:175–86.
13. Toriumi DM. Rhinoplasty: facial plastic surgery: the essential guide. Stuttgart, Germany: Thieme Medical Publishers Inc.; 2005:223–53.
14. Gunter JP, Friedman RM. Lateral crural strut graft: technique and clinical applications in rhinoplasty. Plast Reconstr Surg 1997;99:943–55.
15. Rohrich RJ, Raniere J Jr, Ha RY. The alar contour graft: correction and prevention of alar rim deformities in rhinoplasty. Plast Reconstr Surg 2002;109:2495–505.
16. Kim DW, Toriumi DM. Nasal analysis for secondary rhinoplasty. Facia l Plast Surg Clin North Am 2003;11:399–419.

# Grafting in Rhinoplasty

Michael J. Brenner, MD[a],*, Peter A. Hilger, MD, FACS[b]

**KEYWORDS**

- Rhinoplasty • Graft • Grafting
- Structure • Framework • Cartilage

## PHILOSOPHICAL CONSIDERATIONS

Traditional practice in rhinoplasty has tended to rely on resection of the nasal osseocartilaginous framework to achieve aesthetic or functional objectives. Most successes using this approach have proved short lived because the weakened nasal scaffold remaining after reductive surgery often has inadequate strength to withstand the contractile forces of healing. The classic stigmata of an overresected nose, including alar retraction, internal and external nasal valve collapse, midvault collapse, loss of tip support and projection, and unnatural sharp contours such as bossae formation, have become all too familiar to the revision rhinoplasty surgeon. The loss of structural integrity observed in patients who have saddle nose deformity is frequently an iatrogenic complication caused by failure to preserve an adequate dorsal strut at the time of surgery. The resulting pattern of dorsal and middle vault depression, tip overrotation, loss of tip projection, retraction of the columella, and unnatural contours in these patients is disfiguring and functionally crippling. The poor durability of aesthetic outcomes and the progressive functional impairment associated with reductive surgery have provided a major impetus for the development of grafting approaches in rhinoplasty.

This article details the role of structural and aesthetic grafting in rhinoplasty with the objective of promoting reproducible and durable surgical outcomes. A review of the various grafting materials available to the rhinoplasty surgeon is followed by a discussion of the relevant anatomy, terminology, and indications for each grafting approach. In keeping with the objective of achieving predictable long-term results, emphasis is placed on the use of autogenous cartilage grafts, which are associated with more favorable outcomes and lower complication rates than other, alternative grafting materials.[1,2] This topic alone can justify an independent text, and we are sensitive to the constraints associated with this publication. Therefore, we have provided concise descriptions and illustrations of the relevant surgical techniques and appended a detailed bibliography for readers seeking further discussion.

The soft tissue skin envelope and its underlying osseocartilaginous framework are intimately related, together influencing the external appearance and functionality of the nose.[3] In primary rhinoplasty, suboptimal surgical outcomes commonly result from the buckling of a weakened nasal skeleton that lacks sufficient structural rigidity to withstand the contracture forces generated by the healing soft tissue skin envelope. In revision rhinoplasty, the limiting factor in correcting a previously operated nose is frequently the quality, degree of contraction, and lack of elasticity of the soft tissue skin envelope and the intranasal lining.[4] It is therefore imperative that the surgeon be able to understand and conceptualize the dynamics of postoperative healing while manipulating the nasal framework. Moreover, the surgeon must possess the requisite skill and intellectual dexterity to modify the proposed surgical plan, because distorted anatomy is frequently encountered during surgery. Virtually all techniques designed to provide focal alteration of form or function will have secondary effects in other areas of the nose. The skilled rhinoplasty surgeon anticipates these alterations and adjusts the procedure appropriately.

[a] Division of Otolaryngology–Head & Neck Surgery, Department of Surgery, Southern Illinois University School of Medicine, 747 North Rutledge Street, P.O. Box 19649, Springfield, IL 62794-9649, USA
[b] Division of Facial Plastic and Reconstructive Surgery, Department of Otolaryngology–Head & Neck Surgery, University of Minnesota School of Medicine, 7373 France Avenue South, Minneapolis, MN 55435-4534, USA
* Corresponding author.
*E-mail address:* mjbrenner@gmail.com (M.J. Brenner).

Facial Plast Surg Clin N Am 17 (2009) 91–113
doi:10.1016/j.fsc.2008.09.009
1064-7406/08/$ – see front matter © 2009 Elsevier Inc. All rights reserved.

Conservative resection, framework remodeling, and judicious use of grafts for augmentation comprise the basis for a structural approach to grafting in rhinoplasty.[5] In primary rhinoplasty, major and minor support mechanisms are often weakened by surgical maneuvers. Grafts are used to reconstitute support elements thus compromised and to effect desired changes. In contrast, revision rhinoplasty often involves rebuilding nasal framework in the setting of significant structural deficiency. Excessive resection involving the lower lateral crura, the caudal septum, and the nasal dorsum is often compounded by disruption of other tip support elements. The resulting weakening of the nasal architecture is further exacerbated by scarification of the nasal lining and external soft tissue covering. The surgeon can use appropriately selected grafting techniques to correct problematic anatomy or to protect at-risk areas. A systematic approach to grafting makes it possible to achieve lasting improvement in aesthetic appearance and nasal function, always taking care not to compromise function in the pursuit of aesthetic gain.

## GRAFT MATERIALS

Various grafts and implants are available for use in primary and revision rhinoplasty. Although no ideal grafting material exists, with appropriate graft selection and sound surgical technique, dependable outcomes can be achieved. Grafts can be broadly categorized into autogenous, homologous, and alloplastic types. Injectable agents such as hyaluronic acid fillers are occasionally used for refinements.[6]

### Autogenous Grafts

Autogenous grafts are harvested from the patient and include cartilage, bone, and various soft tissues, such as perichondrium and temporalis fascia. Autogenous cartilage is the structural grafting material of choice because of its ease of carving and reliable long-term outcome, with low rates of infection, resorption, and extrusion.[7–9] Autogenous grafts also avoid the potential risk for an immune response or viral contamination. Cartilage grafts are useful for providing structural scaffolding and creating contour. Representative septal, auricular, and costochondral grafts are shown in **Fig. 1**. When crushed, cartilage remains viable and supports the growth of surrounding cartilage.[10]

Septal cartilage is the most commonly used grafting material in primary rhinoplasty, owing to its straightforward harvest and lack of functional or cosmetic donor site morbidity. Furthermore, septal cartilage is particularly versatile in grafting

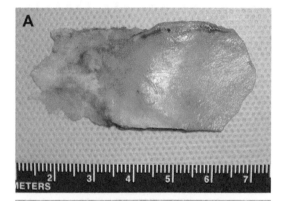

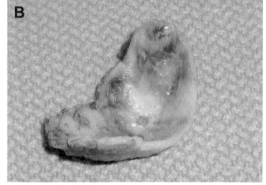

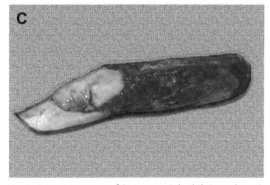

Fig. 1. Autogenous grafting materials. (*A*) Septal cartilage. (*B*) Conchal cartilage. (*C*) Costochondral graft ("floater rib").

and has reliable long-term results. It is useful for spreader grafts, columellar struts, alar battens, dorsal augmentation, and alar rim grafts. Septal cartilage can also be crushed to provide volume augmentation or to soften contour transitions. When harvesting septal cartilage, it is important that a 1.0- to 1.5-cm L-shaped caudal and dorsal strut is maintained. Septal cartilage is often limited in the revision rhinoplasty setting. For major revisions, we prefer to harvest cartilage using an open rhinoplasty approach in which bilateral submucoperiosteal and submucoperichondrial flap elevation is combined with division of the upper lateral cartilages. With this approach, the septum and nasal dorsum are "ouvert au ciel" (open to the sky), achieving unparalleled exposure for diagnosis, harvest of residual structural material, and treatment of structural deformities.

Auricular cartilage is usually harvested for use in revision rhinoplasty when septal cartilage is inadequate. The auricular cartilage is more malleable than septal cartilage and has a curved shape. This curvature and pliability make auricular cartilage a less desirable grafting material for certain purposes, such as when spreader grafts are needed or a thin columellar strut is desired. It is useful to determine preoperatively if one ear is more prominent than the other, because conchal harvest may confer a subtle decrease in the prominence of the donor ear. Alternatively, the surgeon may ask the patient if he or she prefers to sleep on a given side (a "sleep crease" is often discernible in the preauricular region on this side) and then use the contralateral ear. We prefer to harvest auricular cartilage grafts from a postauricular approach because the dissection is straightforward and the incision is hidden. When the conchal bowl is harvested, care is taken to preserve the antihelical fold and a strut of cartilage projecting from the crus helicis, which divides the concha cymba and concha cavum. These measures avoid deformity of the auricle. The soft tissue dead space of the donor site is eliminated by a Betadine ointment bolster that is secured with through-and-through 3-0 nylon sutures. The concha cymba has dimensions, contour, and structural characteristics similar to the lower lateral cartilage, making it a favorable donor site for reconstruction of this structure. Composite grafts from this site may prove particularly useful in the correction of alar retraction. The concha cavum has a concave shape that makes it advantageous for tip grafts, alar battens, and dorsal onlay grafts.

Costochondral grafts afford the rhinoplasty surgeon ample grafting material for the structurally deficient nose. Rib cartilage is most likely to be required either after a disfiguring traumatic injury or following overzealous resection during prior reductive rhinoplasty. The excellent quality and quantity of costal cartilage make this the donor site of choice when septal and auricular cartilage is insufficient. The principal disadvantages of rib cartilage are the tendency for warping, the donor site scar and postoperative pain, the potential for rigidity and calcification of the cartilage in the mature patient, and the added operative time. The patient must also be counseled regarding the small, yet well-established, risks for infection, hematoma, postoperative splinting, and pneumothorax associated with this donor site. We have found the use of continuous infusion anesthetic pumps with 0.25% bupivacaine to be a simple and effective method for managing postoperative pain and decreasing the need for systemic analgesia.

Autogenous bone grafts for rhinoplasty are most useful for grafting of the upper third of the nose and are obtained from the calvarium, the rib, or, less frequently, the iliac crest. Calvarial bone, which is membranous bone, resists resorption and maintains contour more effectively than iliac bone, which is of endochondral origin.[11] Calvarial bone is also associated with less donor site morbidity, although complications of cerebrospinal fluid leakage, sagittal sinus laceration, intracranial injury, and subdural hematoma have been described.[12] Calvarial bone is harvested as a split calvarial bone graft through a hemicoronal incision over the parietal skull. Rib cartilage is much preferred to rib bone grafts. Although autogenous bone grafting is well established in the rhinoplasty literature,[13] we seldom use these donor sites because of susceptibility to fracture, greater difficulty of carving and securing grafts, tendency for a rigid tip or visible graft step-off, and the potential for significant donor site morbidity.

Various other autogenous materials are also useful for soft tissue augmentation in rhinoplasty, principally as adjuncts to structural grafting. Examples include costal perichondrium (collected at the time of costochondral graft harvest), temporalis fascia, and fibroadipose tissue from the postauricular region that can be flattened into a thin sheet with an otologic fascia press. Each of these tissues can be harvested with little or no additional donor site morbidity. These grafts may confer significant aesthetic benefit by softening the framework–soft tissue interface. Most commonly, these tissues are used to camouflage cartilage grafts or to correct minor contour irregularities. In revision rhinoplasty, soft tissue may be used to underlay skin that is thin and atrophic secondary to scarring, contracture, or steroid injection. This soft tissue decreases the risk for graft extrusion, prevents bossae formation, protects the overlying soft tissue skin envelope, and improves the overall quality of the skin envelope.[14] Tragal cartilage or perichondrium may also be used for small grafts.

### Homologous Grafts

The most commonly used homografts are irradiated rib for structural grafting and acellularized dermal matrix for soft tissue augmentation. Historically, these grafts, derived from human cadavers, have proved less predictable than autogenous tissue in their ability to resist resorption and warping; however, experience has been mixed.[15–18] The potential risk for transmission of human pathogens also remains a concern for patients. Nonetheless, these grafting materials are useful in selected patients who are poor candidates for harvest of autogenous tissue or who are unwilling to have an additional donor site. These situations occur only rarely. Costal cartilage homografts are harvested from prescreened cadavers and are subjected to at least 30,000 Gy of radiation to decrease antigenicity. These grafts are associated with low infection and extrusion rates, although soaking in antibiotic solution before use is still recommended. Acellularized dermal matrix has been shown to have significant resorption within the first year, although this tendency for resorption may stabilize thereafter.[19,20] Because of this limitation, acellularized dermal matrix is more appropriately used for graft camouflage and smoothing contour under thin skin than for volume augmentation.

## Alloplasts

In recent years, alloplasts have become more popular because of their relative ease of use, limitless supply, predesigned or easily adaptable shape, and lack of donor site morbidity. Most alloplasts are polymers, which are long chains of molecular subunits. The more commonly used implants include expanded-porous polytetrafluoroethylene (e-PTFE; Gore-Tex),[21] porous high-density polyethylene (PHDPE; Medpor),[22] polyester fiber mesh (Mersilene),[23] and silicone, which is used primarily in Asian patients who have thick skin.[24] The biologic response elicited by the host after use of an allograft is influenced by the chemical composition and the physical characteristics of the graft. The implantation of all alloplasts causes an inflammatory response. In the acute phase, neutrophils and macrophages are recruited, and protein material coats the implant. Fibroblasts deposit collagen, and phagocytosis occurs for implant particles smaller than 60 micrometers; particles larger than 20 micrometers cause macrophage death and secondary release of local inflammatory mediators.[24]

The presence and size of pores influence the tendency for fibrovascular ingrowth and the risk for infection.[25] Alloplasts with pores that are greater than approximately 50 micrometers will exhibit tissue ingrowth, with larger pores supporting correspondingly greater ingrowth. PHDPE has large pores that permit soft tissue and limited bony ingrowth. These PHDPE grafts are difficult to remove, but they are also more resistant to infection.[26] In contrast, e-PTFE has smaller pores, making it more readily removable after implantation. Silicone forms a fibrous capsule without ingrowth and carries a persistent risk for extrusion

throughout the life of the patient. Not all synthetic agents have withstood the test of time. Polyamide mesh (Supramid), which exhibited excessive degradation and resorption in animal models, is now of historic interest only. Polytetrafluoroethylene (Proplast) demonstrated fragmentation with mechanical stress in temporomandibular joint surgery, leading to its removal from the United States market.

## SPECIFIC GRAFTING TECHNIQUES

Many grafting techniques have been described for use in primary and revision rhinoplasty. These techniques are categorized by anatomic site in the discussion that follows. Although the descriptions are intended to reflect common uses of particular grafts, many techniques are versatile and can be adapted to suit the particular deformity encountered. Furthermore, this article covers only the more common grafts used in rhinoplasty. Many of these grafts may be placed by either endonasal or external rhinoplasty approaches. The endonasal approach avoids a columellar scar and may reduce postoperative edema; however, in the severely overresected nose, an external rhinoplasty approach should be considered. The external approach allows for improved diagnosis and is most conducive to reconstructing major framework deficiencies, performing precise graft placement, and correcting asymmetries.

## Grafts of the Nasal Tip

### Columellar struts

The columellar strut provides structural support to the nasal tip and improves tip projection. It has become one of the workhorse grafts in rhinoplasty. As shown in **Fig. 2**, the graft is placed between the paired intermediate and medial crura, using either an endonasal or open rhinoplasty approach. The need for a strong columellar strut is most evident in noses with short, weak, or flared medial and intermediate crura. For endonasal positioning, an incision may be made in the columella, usually caudal to the medial crura.[27] Alternatively, an incision may be made either through a small vertical incision between the medial crura or through the skin of the nasal vestibule and medial crura on one side. When using an open rhinoplasty approach, the graft is sutured to the medial crura. Care should be taken to avoid unintended distortion of the nasal tip contour or the infratip lobule. The graft must be placed short of the domes to avoid excessive prominence with a "unidome" configuration. Preserving a small amount of soft tissue over the nasal spine prevents clicking and displacement of the graft with lip movement. For greater stability, the columellar

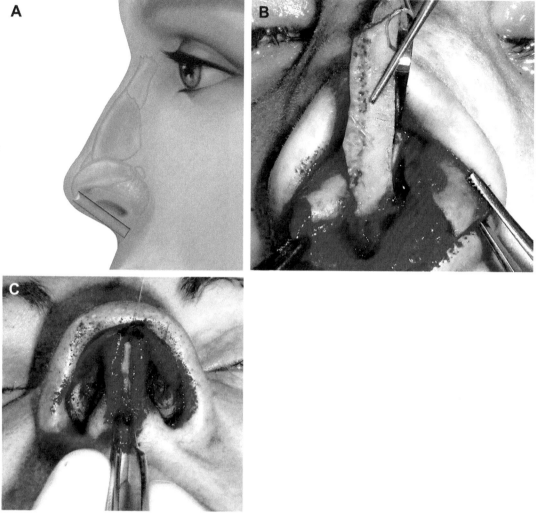

**Fig. 2.** Columellar strut. The columellar strut, one of the "workhorse" grafts of structural rhinoplasty, is placed between the paired intermediate and medial crura. (*A*) Lateral view. (*B*) Placement of graft. (*C*) Columellar strut in position.

strut may be secured to the nasal spine or premaxilla. Septal or costal cartilage is preferable, although double-layered auricular cartilage will often provide sufficient strength. Using the perpendicular plate of the ethmoid or other bone grafts is also effective but requires perforation before suturing. In the patient who has a dependent caudal septum requiring increased projection, establishing a tongue-in-groove relationship between the medial crura and the nasal septum will achieve stability similar to a columellar strut without the need for graft placement.

*Onlay tip grafts*
These grafts are placed over the alar domes as single or multilayer grafts (**Figs. 3** and **4**), using either an endonasal or an external approach.[28]

These grafts are used primarily to camouflage irregularities or to achieve subtle increases in tip projection or contour. Beveling or morselization of the edges minimizes the likelihood of visibility or palpability. The Peck graft (see **Fig. 3**) is a type of onlay tip graft that is made from conchal or septal cartilage. It is classically rectangular and abuts on the domes. The contoured auricular projection graft is a saucer-like disc of cartilage taken from the concha cymba or concha cavum[29] and is useful in rhinoplasty on Asian patients. Cap grafts are classically derived from remnant cartilage after cephalic volume reduction of the lower lateral cartilage (see **Fig. 3**). These cap grafts are small nasal tip grafts used to soften or fill areas of clefting at the nasal tip. They are helpful in improving

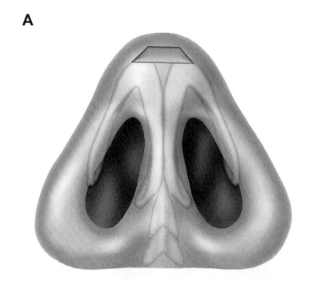

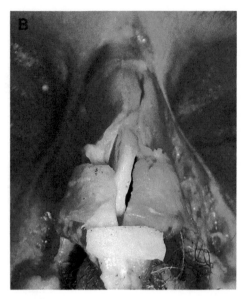

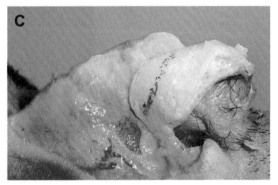

**Fig. 3.** Tip grafting. (*A*) Base view, showing beveled edges of graft that minimize visible edges. (*B*) Peck graft, with its classically rectangular shape. (*C*) Cap graft. Cephalic volume reduction of the lower lateral cartilage provides donor cartilage that may be used as a cap graft of the nasal tip.

the contour of the nasal tip in patients who have thin skin. The graft is placed in the space between the tip-defining points and the medial crura. The term "umbrella graft" is used to describe the use of an onlay tip graft in conjunction with a columellar strut; the columellar strut is the umbrella shaft and the tip onlay graft secured to it forms the top of the umbrella (**Fig. 5**).[30] Placement of tip grafts over the tip-defining points will increase tip projection and definition, whereas placement of these grafts at and below the tip-defining points will increase projection and add volume to the infratip lobule. Whenever possible, it is desirable to stabilize the grafts within a precise pocket. Securing the grafts with fine sutures, particularly with stacked grafts, also minimizes the risk for graft displacement.

### Shield grafts
Shield grafts, sometimes termed Sheen or infra-lobular grafts, are shield-shaped grafts that are positioned over the medial crura, extending from the medial crural footplates to the nasal tip.[31] Examples of these grafts are shown in **Fig. 6**. Initial enthusiasm for these grafts was considerable because of their usefulness in increasing tip projection, defining the nasal tip, and improving the contour of the infratip region. However, the tendency of these grafts to leave a visible "tombstone" impression on the overlying skin subsequently led to much more selective usage. These grafts are best reserved for patients who have thick skin, and the edges should be extensively beveled to minimize visibility. Morselization may be beneficial. The extended shield graft, sometimes termed an "extended columellar strut-tip graft", extends anteriorly beyond the domes to provide added tip projection.[32] In such cases, a small cartilage block placed beneath the graft at the level of the nasal tip may be helpful to increase stability and projection, as shown in **Fig. 6**. These grafts provide the added benefit of

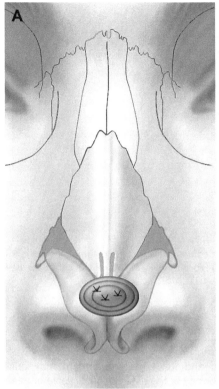

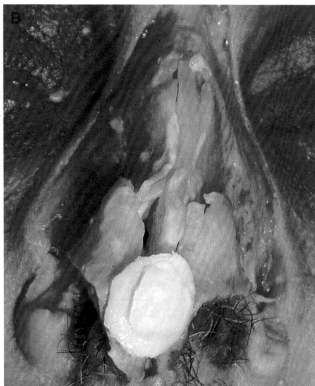

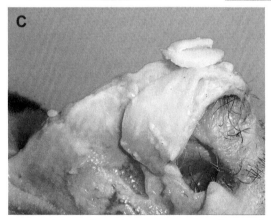

**Fig. 4.** Multilayer tip grafts. Two or more cartilage grafts, usually secured together with suture, may be stacked to achieve greater projection than is possible with a single graft. (*A*) Frontal view. (*B*) Frontal view of tip graft shown in cadaver with soft tissue skin envelope removed. (*C*) Lateral view.

derotation of the overrotated nose. The use of conchal cartilage for this graft improves its pliability and confers a softer contour, thereby decreasing the risk for a visible graft silhouette after resolution of edema.

## Other grafts of the nasal tip

Other, less common, grafts also warrant mention. The anchor graft, so named for its shape, has paired transversely oriented curved wings

(**Fig. 7**). It is carved from auricular cartilage and is used to replace or reinforce the lateral crura, thereby enhancing tip support or projection.[33,34] The subdomal graft, which is placed transversely as a bar under the domes, is used to correct dome asymmetry.[35] It has found application in the correction of the pinched nasal tip and in stabilizing the vertical and horizontal orientation of the domes. Various autogenous materials are useful in softening the appearance of

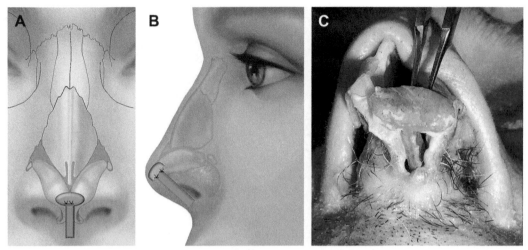

Fig. 5. Umbrella graft. This graft integrates an onlay tip graft with a columellar strut; the columellar strut is the umbrella shaft and the tip onlay graft is the top of the umbrella. (*A*) Frontal view. (*B*) Lateral view. (*C*) Base view of umbrella graft in anatomic position.

cartilaginous grafts and in camouflaging subtle irregularities that may become unmasked in the weeks to months after surgery, as the edema resulting from the operation gradually resolves (**Fig. 8**). Fibroadipose tissue or temporalis fascia are readily harvested from the postauricular region, often at the time of conchal cartilage harvest. Use of perichondrium, crushed cartilage, or connective tissue should always be considered when performing rhinoplasty on patients who have thin skin.

## Grafts of the Alar Region

### Alar batten grafts

Aesthetic and functional impairment may arise from deformity of the external nasal valve or internal nasal valve, or deepening of the alar-nasal groove (**Fig. 9**).[36] Alar batten grafts, shown in **Fig. 10**, are placed in a pocket that extends from the piriform aperture to the paramedian position. The exact position of the graft is determined by the site of maximal collapse. Therefore, the graft

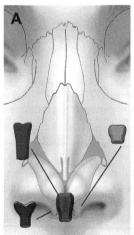
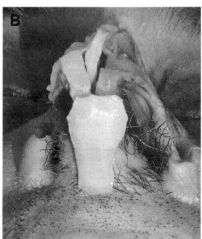
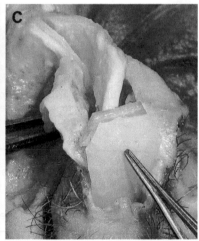

Fig. 6. Shield grafts. Sometimes termed "Sheen" or "infralobular" grafts, these shield-shaped grafts are carved in various shapes and then positioned over the medial crura, extending from the medial crural footplates toward the nasal tip. (*A*) Frontal view, showing examples of various types of shield grafts. (*B*) Base view of shield graft. Note beveling of edges to avoid a visible "tombstone" appearance through skin. (*C*) Extended shield graft with small cartilage block (*green*) to improve stability and projection.

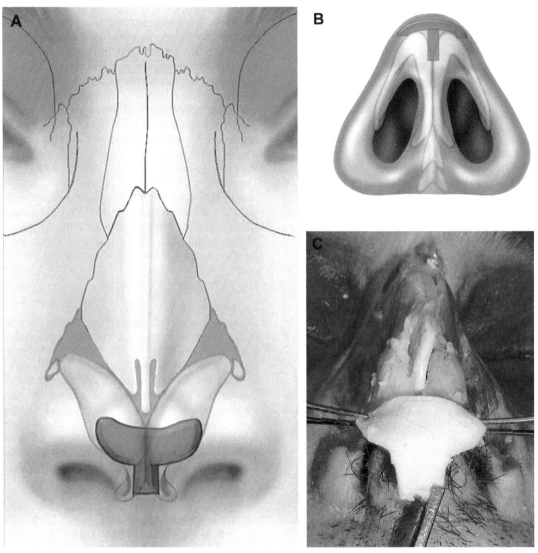

**Fig. 7.** Anchor graft. This modified infratip shield graft, named for its characteristic shape with curved wings, is used to enhance tip projection, improve alar rim position, and augment the infratip region. (*A*) Frontal view. (*B*) Base view. (*C*) Anchor graft shown in cadaver with soft tissue skin envelope removed.

may extend inferior to the caudal aspect of the lateral crus or even toward the alar rim for correction of an overresected lateral crura or external nasal valve collapse. More cephalad positioning allows for treatment of internal nasal valve collapse. Care must be taken with the grafts to avoid creation of a bulbous appearance or visible prominence. In patients who have thin skin, lateral crural strut grafts (discussed below) may be used to achieve improved airway patency with minimal risk for distortion. Auricular cartilage and septal cartilage are most commonly used, although PHDPE grafts are also available.

When placed through an external rhinoplasty approach, we suture fixate the graft to the surface of the lateral crura in at least two locations to ensure adequate stability. Precise pocket preparation is necessary for endonasal placement. In either approach, we routinely place a 5-0 absorbable suture from the vestibular lining, through the lower lateral cartilage in the hinge area, and through the graft and alar skin. A small cutaneous stab incision is then made adjacent to the projecting needle tip to avoid dimpling, and the suture is brought back through the tissues as a simple stitch and tied intranasally.

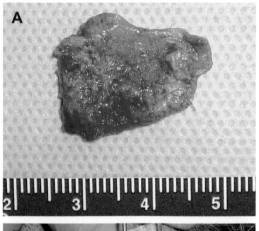

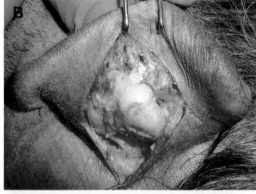

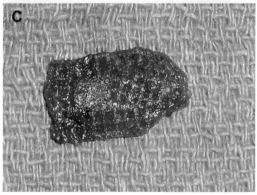

**Fig. 8.** Autogenous camouflage grafts. These grafts can camouflage subtle contour irregularities and soften the appearance of cartilaginous grafts. They are particularly useful in patients who have thin skin. (*A*) Perichondrium. (*B*) Postauricular incision for harvest of conchal cartilage allows access to plentiful fibroadipose tissue. (*C*) Crushed cartilage.

### Alar rim grafts

Alar rim grafts, sometimes referred to as alar contour grafts, are useful in the prevention or correction of alar retraction (**Fig. 11**).[37] These grafts also afford the alae sufficient rigidity to resist collapse, as would otherwise occur in cases of cephalic malposition of the lower lateral cartilages. Additional uses include correction of alar flare and treatment of alar contour irregularity. Cartilaginous alar grafts are nonanatomic grafts that are placed in a subcutaneous pocket immediately above the alar rim. They can be placed through an external rhinoplasty approach, a marginal incision, or a small stab incision just inside the alar margin. Alar rim grafts should be placed so that they do not cross the soft tissue triangle, and the leading edge can be softened to avoid bossae formation. When we place these grafts through an external approach, we stabilize them with a 6-0 absorbable suture anteriorly, thereby avoiding migration superiorly. These grafts are typically capable of achieving 1 to 2 mm of inferior displacement of ala. A large alar batten that extends caudally functions as a combined alar batten and alar rim graft.

### Composite grafts

In cases of severe alar retraction, where a rim graft will not achieve adequate correction, a composite graft is necessary (**Fig. 12**).[38] Composite grafts typically consist of skin, cartilage, and the intervening perichondrium and connective tissue elements. These grafts may be harvested from various locations, including the concha cymba, concha cavum, or auricular root. Usually, the cartilaginous portion of the graft is larger than the overlying skin to maximize the structural augmentation. These grafts are also beneficial in the treatment of vestibular stenosis.

### Lateral crural strut graft

The lateral crural strut graft, shown in **Fig. 13**, is well suited to the thin-skinned patient who has a moderate degree of alar collapse and in whom an unfavorable aesthetic result would be expected with alar batten grafting. Lateral crural strut grafts allow for correction of alar rim collapse, deformed lateral crura, and mild alar retraction.[39] These grafts, like alar batten grafts, are effective for straightening the lateral crus, especially when recurvature of the lower lateral crura is present. These grafts are also useful in providing support to the nasal tip when cephalic malposition is present and the alae must be repositioned. These grafts require dissection of the vestibular skin from the undersurface of the lower lateral cartilage and are placed between the lateral crus and the vestibular skin. The lateral aspect of the rim graft is usually positioned superficial to the piriform aperture and caudal to the alar groove. Although extremely useful, these grafts are more technically difficult than batten grafts. They also tend to

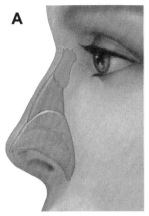
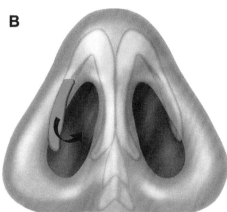
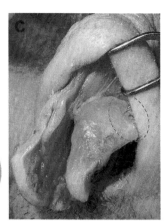

**Fig. 9.** Sites of nasal collapse. (*A*) Internal and external nasal valve collapse occurs in the purple region, which spans the lower third of the nose and caudal aspect of the nasal midvault, including the hinge area. Alar batten grafts can be placed anywhere in this region. The midvault (*blue region*) is classically stented with spreader grafts. Nasal bones (*green*) denote upper third of nose. (*B*) Recurvature of the lower lateral crura (*green*) narrows the nasal airway and can be corrected with cartilaginous grafting. (*C*) Collapse at hinge area on cadaveric specimen is denoted by the broken line ellipse.

protrude slightly into the nasal airway and impart less structural rigidity than alar batten grafts.

### Other grafts of the alar region

Several other, less common, alar grafts have also been described. The lateral crural spanning graft, also referred to as an alar spreader graft, is a transverse graft that spans the intercrural space (**Fig. 14**).[40] This graft allows for correction or prevention of an overly narrowed or pinched nasal tip. It is secured to both lateral crura for stabilization and must be beveled to avoid being discernable postoperatively. These grafts may make the tip more bulbous if not carefully contoured. Lateral crural turnover grafts are used to create thicker and stronger lateral crura. Longitudinal scoring or partial-thickness incision along the undersurface of the lateral crura is followed by suturing of the cephalic portion of the lateral crura to its caudal remnant.[41] The lateral crural onlay graft is used to strengthen and shape alae that are weakened or have irregular contour. The grafts are placed over the lateral crus to improve external nasal valve function. This graft has some similarity to the alar batten graft, although it more closely mirrors alar cartilage anatomy. Care must be taken to bevel these grafts so as to avoid a "step-off" deformity.

### Grafts of the Nasal Dorsum and Midvault

#### Spreader grafts (and extended spreader grafts)

Spreader grafts, shown in **Fig. 15**, are longitudinally oriented grafts, usually paired, that are secured deep to the mucoperichondrium between the nasal septum and upper lateral cartilages. These grafts are among the most commonly used and versatile grafts in both primary and revision rhinoplasty. They are frequently used to reconstruct an open roof deformity and to smooth the brow–tip aesthetic line. Spreader grafts prevent or correct midvault collapse by stenting open the internal nasal valve, thereby avoiding medial displacement of the upper lateral cartilages.[42] Occasionally, grafts with asymmetric width are helpful in managing pre-existing midvault irregularities. We usually place these grafts through an external approach to facilitate suture fixation after the upper lateral cartilages and septum are separated. We seldom place spreader grafts beneath intact lower lateral cartilages because this method produces less reliable outcomes.

Several adaptations to the spreader grafts have been described. The term "pistol grafts" refers to spreader grafts that extend above the dorsal septum to augment the dorsum. When performing this maneuver, it is important to appropriately camouflage the irregularity that is produced. When spreader grafts project caudally to lengthen the nose or increase tip projection, they are referred to as extended spreader grafts or septal extension grafts.[43] The caudal ends of the grafts are sutured to the medial surfaces of the intermediate crura of the lower lateral cartilages, thereby providing tip derotation. The dynamic adjustable rotational tip (DART) grafts are long spreader grafts used to correct tip deprojection and overrotation in patients who have overly resected, weakened cartilage frameworks.[44] Spreader grafts may also extend

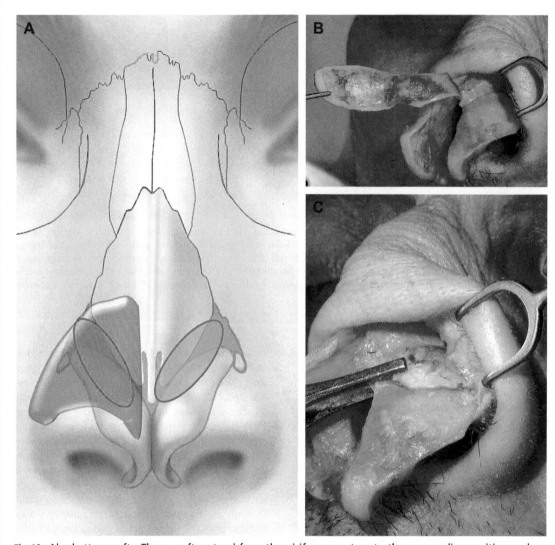

**Fig. 10.** Alar batten grafts. These grafts extend from the piriform aperture to the paramedian position and are positioned at the site of maximal collapse. (*A*) Frontal view showing standard position of alar batten grafts in blue. Purple indicates the larger range of possible placement for these grafts, depending on the site of collapse. (*B*) Three-quarter view showing a large alar batten graft carved from auricular conchal cartilage. The graft convexity will promote nasal airway patency. (*C*) Graft in position.

cephalically to slightly widen the bony nasal pyramid, although widening at this site is only occasionally indicated.

### Septal extension grafts and septal replacement grafts

Septal extension grafts include various grafts that are used to enhance nasal tip dynamics by building stable framework onto the existing septal scaffold.[45,46] The size and position of septal extension grafts are varied to influence projection, to derotate the tip, or to fill out the columella-labial angle, thereby suggesting tip rotation. Some septal extension grafts are actually long spreader grafts

that span from the nasal septum, beyond the anterior septal angle, and into the interdomal region (**Fig. 16**). A second type of septal extension graft involves cartilage grafts that run diagonally from the septal angle to the tip–lobule complex. The third type of graft, sometimes termed a "caudal septal extension graft", is a direct extension from the caudal septum that can control the projection, rotation, and strength of the tip (**Fig. 17**). This graft confers considerable strength and stability because of its rigid foundation. The medial crura can be repositioned along this augmented septum, and lateral crural steal may be used to optimize tip projection. In cases in which a caudal

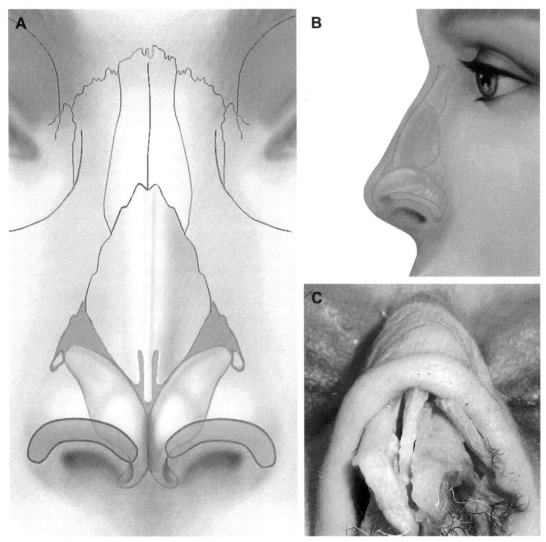

**Fig. 11.** Alar rim grafts. Also referred to as alar contour grafts, these grafts are used to correct alar retraction and to provide support to the external nasal valve. (*A*) Frontal view. (*B*) Lateral view. (*C*) Alar rim graft in anatomic position.

septum is weak or missing, resulting in alar-columellar disproportion, a septal extension graft or caudal septal replacement graft (**Fig. 18**) will improve tip support and correct columellar retraction.[47]

### Dorsal onlay graft

The dorsal onlay graft, shown in **Fig. 19**, is used to correct minor and major deformities of the nasal dorsum. Commonly, we design these grafts to span the entire length of the nasal dorsum, from the radix to the septal angle, to minimize the risk for palpable irregularities.[7] Smaller refinement grafts may be used as beveled or crushed grafts to address contour irregularities or asymmetries. Although septal or conchal cartilage is usually

sufficient for refinement of the nasal dorsum, costal cartilage is indicated in those cases where major augmentation is required. Examples include severe saddle nose deformity, traumatic compressive fractures, or other major structural deficits. Alternatives are e-PTFE, PHDPE, and silicone (in patients who have thick skin), although autogenous material is preferred. If e-PTFE is used, we avoid dissection that communicates to dorsal and septal surgical sites because we believe that doing so increases the risk for alloplast infection.

We routinely harvest a "floater" rib, which is straighter and less prone to warping than the sixth or seventh rib. This floater rib is harvested as half bone and half cartilage, thereby mirroring the natural osseocartilaginous anatomy of the nasal

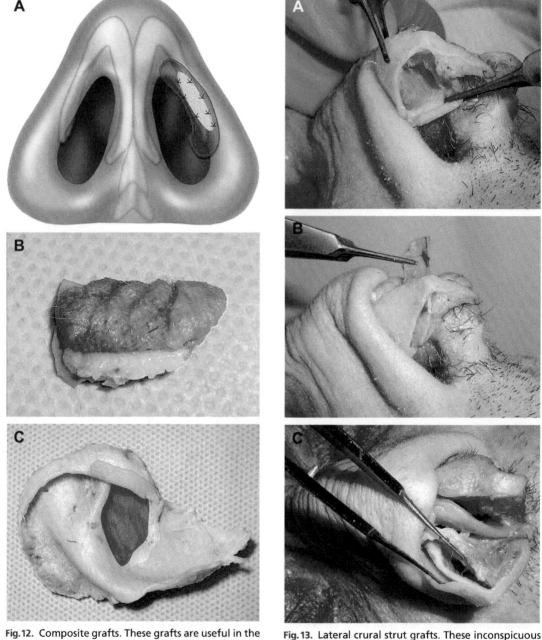

Fig. 12. Composite grafts. These grafts are useful in the treatment of vestibular stenosis and correction of severe alar retraction not amenable to rim grafting. (*A*) Base view shows composite graft in nasal vestibule. Note that the structural cartilaginous component of the graft (*green*) is larger than the overlying skin component (*stippled pink*). (*B*) Composite graft. (*C*) Auricular cartilage showing common sites of graft harvest, including concha cymba (*red*), concha cavum (*blue*), and auricular root (*green*).

Fig. 13. Lateral crural strut grafts. These inconspicuous grafts are placed deep to the alar cartilage and allow for correction of moderate alar collapse, lower lateral cartilage recurvature, and mild alar retraction. (*A*) Vestibular lining is dissected away from the undersurface of the lower lateral cartilage, creating a pocket for graft placement. (*B*) Placement of graft. (*C*) Lateral crural strut graft in anatomic position.

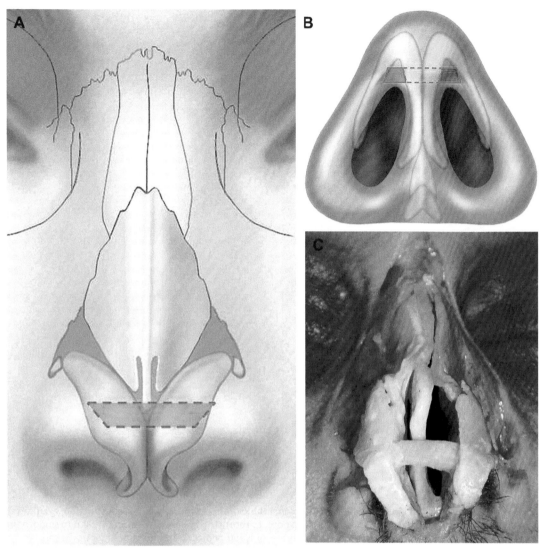

**Fig. 14.** Lateral crural spanning graft. Also referred to as an alar spreader graft, this graft allows for correction of an overly narrowed or pinched nasal tip. (*A*) Frontal view. (*B*) Base view. (*C*) Graft shown in anatomic position.

dorsum. The bony portion of the graft is positioned cephalically, and the undersurface is carved in a gently curving concave contour to ensure that the graft will be seated firmly and to expose the cancellous trabecular bone. Before securing the graft, the surgeon then rasps down the bony foundation where the graft will sit until punctuate bleeding is encountered. The contact of raw bone to raw bone thus achieved promotes effective osseointegration of the cantilevered graft to the underlying bony foundation. The dorsal onlay graft obviates the need for spreader grafts because the upper lateral cartilages are sutured to the lateral cartilaginous aspects of the graft. The graft is then rigidly fixated with a percutaneous Kirschner wire (K-wire) that further promotes rigid

fixation and minimizes the risk for warping.[48] The K-wire is easily removed in the office in 3 weeks.

Rarely, it is necessary to articulate the dorsal graft and a columellar strut. This approach is most useful when a profound loss of structural support in the lower third of the nose occurs. For example, in patients who have significant saddle deformity, the lower third of the nose is usually poorly supported, and a strong cartilaginous columellar strut is required, along with an integrated cartilaginous premaxillary graft. The columellar strut and premaxillary graft are placed through an open rhinoplasty approach with dissection between the medial crura. The premaxillary graft is fixated with a percutaneous K-wire.

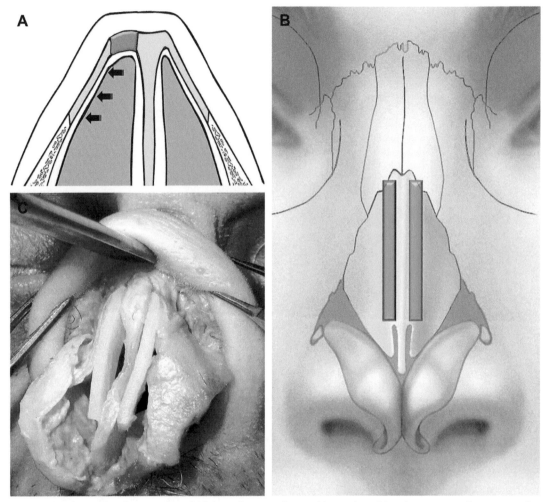

**Fig. 15.** Spreader grafts. These grafts, which have become the workhorse for midvault reconstruction, are used to correct or prevent collapse of the middle third of the nose, to reconstruct open roof deformity, and to smooth the brow-tip aesthetic line. (*A*) This axial section through the midvault demonstrates how spreader grafts can expand the nasal airway. (*B*) Frontal view. (*C*) Spreader grafts in anatomic position.

### Skoog technique modification

In patients who have short nasal bones and long upper lateral cartilages, a modification of the Skoog technique for dorsal reduction may be advantageous (**Fig. 20**). In this procedure, the osseocartilaginous dorsal convexity is removed as a unit, the underlying nasal dorsum is reduced, and the osseocartilaginous unit is then sculpted by shaving off the residual septal remnant on the undersurface and replaced in it is original anatomic location. The upper lateral cartilages are subsequently secured to this anatomic osseocartilaginous graft with suture fixation. This approach is attractive from aesthetic and functional aspects because it accomplishes dorsal reduction,

correction of the open roof deformity, preservation of the middle vault, and restoration of the natural contouring of the nasal dorsum while obviating the need for osteotomies.[49]

### Radix graft

Radix grafts, shown in **Fig. 21**, are used to reposition the radix in a more cephalic and anterior position. This maneuver provides the perception of lengthening the nose and can also be used to augment an inadequate nasofrontal angle.[50] Precise subperiosteal pocket preparation minimizes the risk for graft displacement. The grafts may be single or layered, and beveling or crushing of the sides of the grafts will decrease perceptibility.

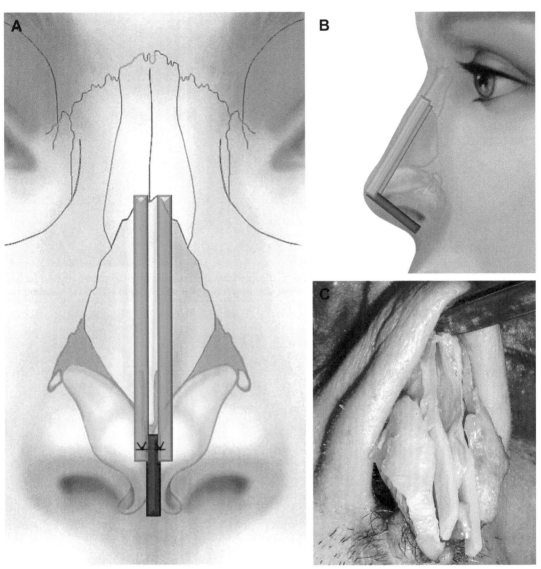

Fig.16. DART grafts stabilized with columellar strut. These elongated spreader grafts extend into the dome as septal extension grafts and can increase projection and derotate the tip. Stability is optimized when they are integrated with a columellar strut, as depicted in these figures. (*A*) Frontal view. (*B*) Lateral view. (*C*) Grafts in anatomic position.

Deficiency of the radix is easily overlooked and may prompt excessive resection of the nasal dorsum if the dorsum is brought down to the level of the radix. Significant iatrogenic deformity can result from this error in judgment. Thoughtful application of this simple, yet powerful, grafting technique can yield satisfying results. The aesthetic perception of nasal lengthening achieved with this graft, although limited, is far more predictable than the lengthening achieved by stretching

the soft tissue skin envelope and increasing projection. Furthermore, the radix graft does not pose the risk for introducing asymmetry or other deformity to the lower third of the nose.[50]

## Lateral nasal wall grafts

Lateral nasal wall grafts, also referred to as dorsal sidewall onlay grafts, are grafts of variable size that are used to correct focal depression or contour irregularity along the lateral nose.[51] The grafts are

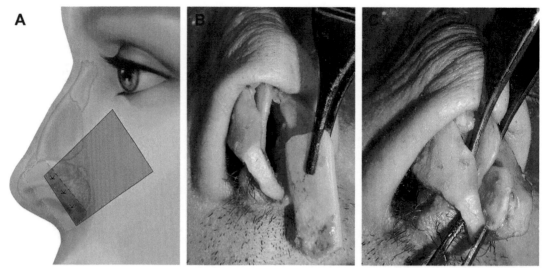

**Fig. 17.** Caudal septal extension graft. This graft extends directly from the caudal septum to control the projection, rotation, and strength of the nasal tip. (*A*) Lateral view, showing columellar strut (*green*) secured to nasal septum (*red*). (*B*) Placement of graft. (*C*) Graft in anatomic position.

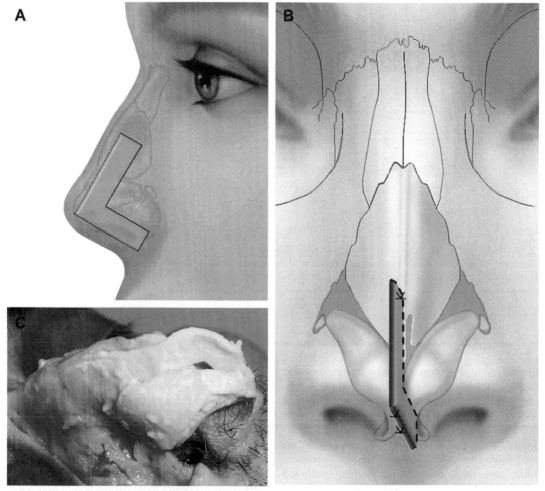

**Fig. 18.** Caudal septal replacement graft. This graft is useful when the caudal septum is weak, deformed, or absent. (*A*) Lateral view. (*B*) Frontal view. (*C*) Graft in anatomic position.

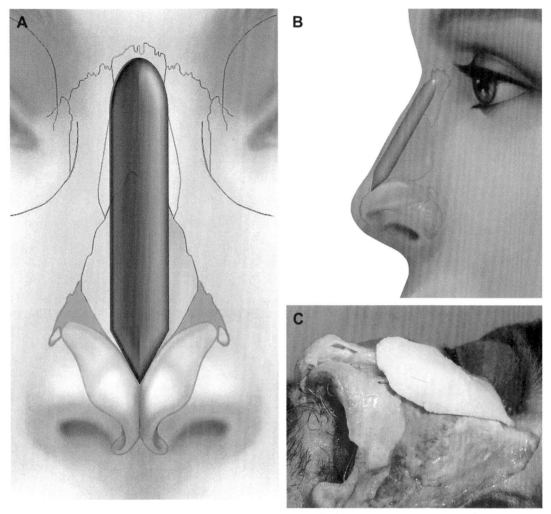

Fig. 19. Dorsal onlay graft. Septal and auricular cartilage are useful for improving the contour of the nasal dorsum, whereas costal cartilage is indicated in cases where major augmentation is required, as in severe saddle nose deformity. (*A*) Frontal view. (*B*) Lateral view. (*C*) Graft shown in cadaver with soft tissue skin envelope removed.

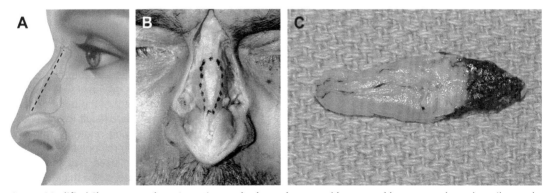

Fig. 20. Modified Skoog procedure. In patients who have short nasal bones and long upper lateral cartilages, the osseocartilaginous dorsal convexity is removed and sculpted for use as a dorsal onlay graft after appropriate reduction of the underlying nasal dorsum. (*A*) Dashed line denotes osseocartilaginous convexity to be removed with scalpel and Rubin osteotome. (*B*) Cadaveric demonstration of regions to be sculpted into onlay graft. (*C*) Sculpted onlay graft showing short nasal bones and long cartilaginous component.

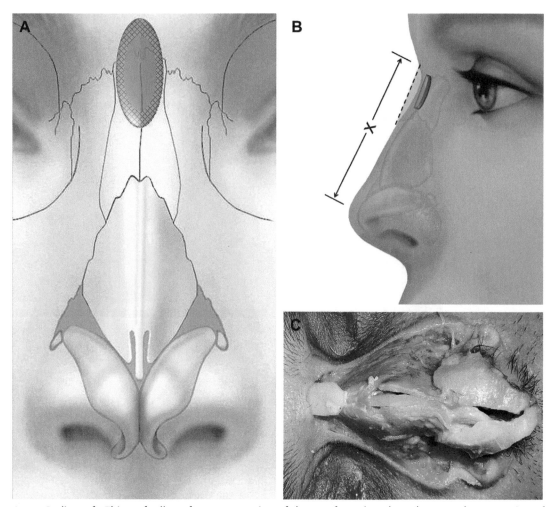

**Fig. 21.** Radix graft. This graft allows for augmentation of the nasofrontal angle and creates the perception of nasal lengthening by repositioning the radix. (*A*) Frontal view, with peripheral aspect of cartilaginous graft crushed (*crosshatches*) to minimize visibility. (*B*) Lateral view. Green shading and broken line indicate radix being repositioned in a more cephalic and anterior position, thereby increasing nasal length, denoted by "X." (*C*) Graft shown in cadaver with soft tissue skin envelope removed.

positioned along the lateral aspect of the nose in the area of asymmetry and tend to be most useful in the midvault region. The grafts may be crushed or rigid, although rigid grafts are more likely to be discernible when placed over the bony pyramid of the upper third of the nose. When a cosmetic deformity of the midvault is associated with nasal airway obstruction, either spreader grafts or another grafting technique that simultaneously addresses the functional problem should be used.

## Grafts of the Premaxilla and Alar Base

### Columellar plumping grafts
Columellar plumping grafts, shown in **Fig. 22**, consist of diced or morselized cartilage that is placed at the posterior aspect of the columella. Placing graft material in the region between the nasal spine

and medial crural footplates results in widening of the columellar-labial angle. This graft thus creates an appearance of nasal tip rotation.[52]

### Premaxillary grafting
The premaxillary graft is used to augment an underdeveloped or retrusive premaxilla. It involves grafting of the caudal aspect of the piriform aperture.[52] These grafts may be difficult to carve and, depending on the underlying anatomy, may require substantial volume. In rhinoplasty in Asians, silicone implants are often used and thought to be better tolerated because of the thicker skin in this ethnic population.[53,54] Costal cartilage is another option well suited to this location, particularly if the use of costal cartilage for another part of the reconstruction is already indicated.

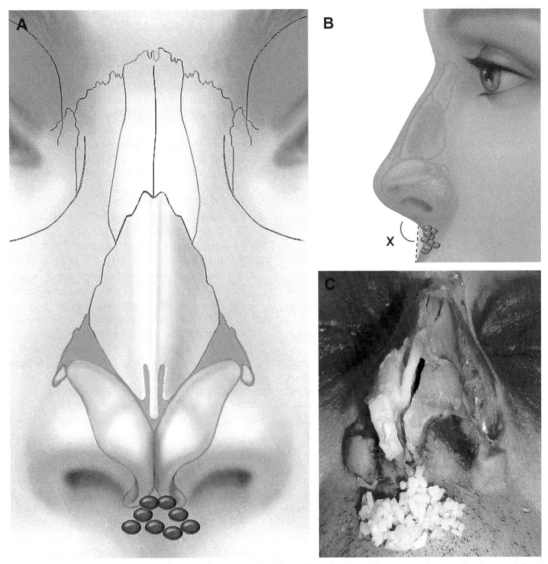

**Fig. 22.** Columellar plumping grafts. Diced or morselized cartilage is placed between the nasal spine and foot-plates of the medial crura to widen the columellar-labial angle. This technique creates the illusion of tip rotation. (*A*) Frontal view. (*B*) Lateral view. Green shading and broken line indicated widening of the columellar-labial angle, X°. (*C*) The plumping grafts, shown in figure, are placed subcutaneously.

## *Alar base grafts*

Alar base grafts are used along the lateral piriform aperture to augment a posteriorly displaced interface of the lip and ala.[55] The alar base composite graft is particularly useful in reconstruction of the cleft lip nasal deformity. This deformity exemplifies how the lack of a stable platform in the premaxilla precludes a normal relationship between the lip and nose. In cases of significant bony deficiency of the premaxilla, a corticocancellous bone graft may be necessary to reconstruct the underlying deformity.

## SUMMARY

The development of sophisticated grafting techniques has played an integral role in achieving durable surgical outcomes in rhinoplasty. The loss of structural integrity often encountered after reductive rhinoplasty illustrates the importance of preservation of framework. The structural approach to rhinoplasty uses grafts to maintain and augment nasal support mechanisms and in doing so, enables the nasal skeleton to resist contractile forces of healing that would otherwise compromise aesthetic and functional results.

## ACKNOWLEDGMENTS

The authors wish to thank Eric Dobratz, MD, for his assistance with the laboratory dissections used for selected figures in this publication.

## REFERENCES

1. Adamson PA. Grafts in rhinoplasty: autogenous grafts are superior to alloplastic. Arch Otolaryngol Head Neck Surg 2000;126(4):561–2.
2. Toriumi DM. Autogenous grafts are worth the extra time. Arch Otolaryngol Head Neck Surg 2000;126(4):562–4.
3. Quatela VC, Jacono AA. Structural grafting in rhinoplasty. Facial Plast Surg 2002;18(4):223–32.
4. Toriumi DM, Patel AB, Derosa J. Correcting the short nose in revision rhinoplasty. Facial Plast Surg Clin North Am 2006;14(4):343–55.
5. Whitaker EG, Johnson CM Jr. The evolution of open structure rhinoplasty. Arch Facial Plast Surg 2003; 5(4):291–300.
6. Biesman B. Soft tissue augmentation using Restylane. Facial Plast Surg 2004;20(2):171–7.
7. Gunter JP, Rohrich RJ. Augmentation rhinoplasty: dorsal onlay grafting using shaped autogenous septal cartilage. Plast Reconstr Surg 1990;86(1):39–45.
8. Ortiz-Monasterio F, Olmedo A, Oscoy LO. The use of cartilage grafts in primary aesthetic rhinoplasty. Plast Reconstr Surg 1981;67(5):597–605.
9. Tardy ME Jr, Denneny J III, Fritsch MH. The versatile cartilage autograft in reconstruction of the nose and face. Laryngoscope 1985;95(5):523–33.
10. Cakmak O, Bircan S, Buyuklu F, et al. Viability of crushed and diced cartilage grafts: a study in rabbits. Arch Facial Plast Surg 2005;7(1):21–6.
11. Smith JD, Abramson M. Membranous vs endochondrial bone autografts. Arch Otolaryngol 1974;99(3):203–5.
12. Frodel JL Jr, Marentette LJ, Quatela VC, et al. Calvarial bone graft harvest. Techniques, considerations, and morbidity. Arch Otolaryngol Head Neck Surg 1993;119(1):17–23.
13. Romo T III, Jablonski RD. Nasal reconstruction using split calvarial grafts. Otolaryngol Head Neck Surg 1992;107(5):622–30.
14. Guerrerosantos J. Nose and paranasal augmentation: autogenous, fascia, and cartilage. Clin Plast Surg 1991;18(1):65–86.
15. Adams WP Jr, Rohrich RJ, Gunter JP, et al. The rate of warping in irradiated and nonirradiated homograft rib cartilage: a controlled comparison and clinical implications. Plast Reconstr Surg 1999;103(1):265–70.
16. Dingman RO, Grabb WC. Costal cartilage homografts preserved by irradiation. Plast Reconstr Surg Transplant Bull 1961;28:562–7.
17. Song HM, Lee BJ, Jang YJ. Processed costal cartilage homograft in rhinoplasty: the Asian Medical Center experience. Arch Otolaryngol Head Neck Surg 2008;134(5):485–9.
18. Strauch B, Wallach SG. Reconstruction with irradiated homograft costal cartilage. Plast Reconstr Surg 2003;111(7):2405–11.
19. Gryskiewicz JM, Rohrich RJ, Reagan BJ. The use of AlloDerm for the correction of nasal contour deformities. Plast Reconstr Surg 2001;107(2): 561–70.
20. Sclafani AP, Romo T III, Jacono AA, et al. Evaluation of acellular dermal graft (AlloDerm) sheet for soft tissue augmentation: a 1-year follow-up of clinical observations and histological findings. Arch Facial Plast Surg 2001;3(2):101–3.
21. Conrad K, Torgerson CS, Gillman GS. Applications of GORE-TEX implants in rhinoplasty reexamined after 17 years. Arch Facial Plast Surg 2008;10(4):224–31.
22. Turegun M, Acarturk TO, Ozturk S, et al. Aesthetic and functional restoration using dorsal saddle shaped Medpor implant in secondary rhinoplasty. Ann Plast Surg 2008;60(6):600–3.
23. Colton JJ, Beekhuis GJ. Use of mersilene mesh in nasal augmentation. Facial Plast Surg 1992;8(3):149–56.
24. Romo T III, Kwak ES. Nasal grafts and implants in revision rhinoplasty. Facial Plast Surg Clin North Am 2006;14(4):373–87.
25. Sclafani AP, Romo T III. Biology and chemistry of facial implants. Facial Plast Surg 2000;16(1):3–6.
26. Sclafani AP, Thomas JR, Cox AJ, et al. Clinical and histologic response of subcutaneous expanded polytetrafluoroethylene (Gore-Tex) and porous high-density polyethylene (Medpor) implants to acute and early infection. Arch Otolaryngol Head Neck Surg 1997;123(3):328–36.
27. Anderson JR. A new approach to rhinoplasty. Trans Am Acad Ophthalmol Otolaryngol 1966;70(2):183–92.
28. Peck GC. The onlay graft for nasal tip projection. Plast Reconstr Surg 1983;71(1):27–39.
29. Porter JP, Tardy ME Jr, Cheng J. The contoured auricular projection graft for nasal tip projection. Arch Facial Plast Surg 1999;1(4):312–5.
30. Peck GC Jr, Michelson L, Segal J, et al. An 18-year experience with the umbrella graft in rhinoplasty. Plast Reconstr Surg 1998;102(6):2158–65.
31. Sheen JH. Achieving more nasal tip projection by the use of a small autogenous vomer or septal cartilage graft. A preliminary report. Plast Reconstr Surg 1975;56(1):35–40.
32. Pastorek NJ, Bustillo A, Murphy MR, et al. The extended columellar strut-tip graft. Arch Facial Plast Surg 2005;7(3):176–84.
33. Chang CW, Davis RE. The anchor graft: a novel technique in rhinoplasty. Arch Facial Plast Surg 2008;10(1):50–5.
34. Juri J, Juri C, Grilli DA, et al. Correction of the secondary nasal tip and of alar and/or columellar collapse. Plast Reconstr Surg 1988;82(1):160–5.

35. Guyuron B, Poggi JT, Michelow BJ. The subdomal graft. Plast Reconstr Surg 2004;113(3):1037–40.

36. Toriumi DM, Josen J, Weinberger M, et al. Use of alar batten grafts for correction of nasal valve collapse. Arch Otolaryngol Head Neck Surg 1997; 123(8):802–8.

37. Rohrich RJ, Raniere J Jr, Ha RY. The alar contour graft: correction and prevention of alar rim deformities in rhinoplasty. Plast Reconstr Surg 2002;109(7):2495–505.

38. Constantian MB. Indications and use of composite grafts in 100 consecutive secondary and tertiary rhinoplasty patients: introduction of the axial orientation. Plast Reconstr Surg 2002;110(4):1116–33.

39. Gunter JP, Friedman RM. Lateral crural strut graft: technique and clinical applications in rhinoplasty. Plast Reconstr Surg 1997;99(4):943–52.

40. Gunter JP, Rohrich RJ. Correction of the pinched nasal tip with alar spreader grafts. Plast Reconstr Surg 1992;90(5):821–9.

41. McCollough EG, Fedok FG. The lateral crural turnover graft: correction of the concave lateral crus. Laryngoscope 1993;103(4 Pt 1):463–9.

42. Sheen JH, Sheen JH. Spreader graft: a method of reconstructing the roof of the middle nasal vault following rhinoplasty. Plast Reconstr Surg 1984;73(2):230–9.

43. Palacin JM, Bravo FG, Zeky R, et al. Controlling nasal length with extended spreader grafts: a reliable technique in primary rhinoplasty. Aesthetic Plast Surg 2007;31(6):645–50.

44. Dyer WK, Yune ME. Structural grafting in rhinoplasty. Facial Plast Surg 1997;13(4):269–77.

45. Byrd HS, Andochick S, Copit S, et al. Septal extension grafts: a method of controlling tip projection shape. Plast Reconstr Surg 1997;100(4):999–1010.

46. Ha RY, Byrd HS. Septal extension grafts revisited: 6-year experience in controlling nasal tip projection and shape. Plast Reconstr Surg 2003;112(7):1929–35.

47. Kridel RW, Chiu RJ. The management of alar columellar disproportion in revision rhinoplasty. Facial Plast Surg Clin North Am 2006;14(4):313–29.

48. Gunter JP, Clark CP, Friedman RM. Internal stabilization of autogenous rib cartilage grafts in rhinoplasty: a barrier to cartilage warping. Plast Reconstr Surg 1997;100(1):161–9.

49. Hall JA, Peters MD, Hilger PA. Modification of the Skoog dorsal reduction for preservation of the middle nasal vault. Arch Facial Plast Surg 2004;6(2):105–10.

50. Becker DG, Pastorek NJ. The radix graft in cosmetic rhinoplasty. Arch Facial Plast Surg 2001;3(2):115–9.

51. Constantian MB. An algorithm for correcting the asymmetrical nose. Plast Reconstr Surg 1989;83(5):801–11.

52. Gunter JP, Landecker A, Cochran CS. Frequently used grafts in rhinoplasty: nomenclature and analysis. Plast Reconstr Surg 2006;118(1):14e–29e.

53. Deva AK, Merten S, Chang L. Silicone in nasal augmentation rhinoplasty: a decade of clinical experience. Plast Reconstr Surg 1998;102(4):1230–7.

54. Lam SM, Kim YK. Augmentation rhinoplasty of the Asian nose with the "bird" silicone implant. Ann Plast Surg 2003;51(3):249–56.

55. Pessa JE, Peterson ML, Thompson JW, et al. Pyriform augmentation as an ancillary procedure in facial rejuvenation surgery. Plast Reconstr Surg 1999;103(2):683–6.

# Functional Rhinoplasty

David W. Kim, MD[a,b,*], Krista Rodriguez-Bruno, MD[a]

**KEYWORDS**

- Functional rhinoplasty • Internal nasal valve
- External nasal valve • Upper lateral cartilages
- Lower lateral cartilages

Over the past couple of decades, there has been an increasingly sophisticated understanding of the pathophysiology underlying fixed nasal obstruction. In the past, submucous resection of the quadrangular cartilage, septoplasty, and inferior turbinate reduction procedures were the predominant workhorse techniques to address fixed nasal obstruction. Although these procedures continue to be a vital part of nasal airway surgery, they do not directly address other types of anatomic obstruction, such as insufficiency of the lateral nasal wall, pinching of the upper lateral cartilage (ULC), or alar collapse. Problems in these areas are part of the large group of disorders lumped into the term "nasal valve insufficiency." To treat these problems, surgeons have adopted a greater range of operative techniques. Taken together, various combinations of these procedures are often described as "functional rhinoplasty." Of note, the methods used within a functional rhinoplasty procedure may vary considerably among different surgeons.

This article reviews the common surgical maneuvers used to treat the various types of fixed nasal obstruction. By way of introduction, the anatomy, pathophysiology, and assessment of the anatomically obstructed nose are reviewed. Outcomes and efficacy of traditional nasal airway procedures are then discussed. Next, surgical techniques, nuances, and pitfalls for the treatment of the internal nasal valve area are detailed. Finally, alternative techniques used to treat the nasal valve areas are briefly reviewed.

## BACKGROUND AND SIGNIFICANCE

Functional and aesthetic rhinoplasties are intimately related. This has become even more evident in the last 20 years, during which the field of facial plastic surgery has experienced an evolution in its surgical philosophy. Previously, emphasis had been placed on reductive techniques that achieved short-term, cosmetic goals, often used at the expense of nasal framework stability. With expanded understanding of the structural and dynamic roles of the nasal scaffold, an increased appreciation has developed for the consequences that surgical modifications have on dynamic nasal airflow.[1,2] Toriumi and coworkers[3] exemplified this trend and focused on a conservative surgical approach aimed at stabilizing and reorienting the nasal anatomic structures instead of reducing them, to ensure long-term cosmetic results while respecting and optimizing nasal airway function.

Functional and aesthetic complaints frequently overlap and the facial plastic surgeon is in a unique position optimally to address both. One of the most common patient grievances seen in many otolaryngology practices is nasal obstruction. Despite the frequency of such a problem, the task of identifying the nasal structures that contribute to the obstruction is not always straightforward.[4] Nasal septal abnormalities are often identified during physical examination, with an estimated 75% to 80% of adults exhibiting some degree of septal deviation.[5] This can mislead physicians who may focus their attention on this finding when planning their surgical approach. Some cases are clear-cut with prominent septal convexities that can be easily targeted surgically. In these patients, a septoplasty may be performed, which in several studies has been shown to be effective.[6-9] Recently, Stewart and colleagues[6] showed that patients with at least moderate septal deviation on examination reported a significant

[a] Department of Otolaryngology, Head and Neck Surgery, University of California, San Francisco, CA, USA
[b] Division of Facial Plastic and Reconstructive Surgery, University of California, San Francisco, CA, USA
* Corresponding author. University of California, Box 1809, 2330 Post Street, San Francisco, CA 94143–1809.
*E-mail address:* dkim@ohns.ucsf.edu (D.W. Kim).

Facial Plast Surg Clin N Am 17 (2009) 115–131
doi:10.1016/j.fsc.2008.09.011
1064-7406/08/$ – see front matter © 2009 Published by Elsevier Inc.

improvement in nasal obstruction after septoplasty surgery, which persisted at 6 months. In a systematic review of the literature, Singh and colleagues[10] found septoplasty to benefit approximately 75% of patients with nasal obstruction.

Many patients exhibit a lesser degree of nasal septal deviation, however, and yet continue to have severe obstructive nasal symptoms. Most typically, this happens as a result of the nasal valves contributing to the obstruction, a process that only is evident during dynamic nasal inspiration. The internal valve is defined as the area between the caudal end of the ULC and the cartilaginous septum including the circumferential neighboring structures in the nasal airway. Narrowing at this location can cause difficulty with air flow. External valve insufficiency is caused by narrowing or weakness of the vestibular nasal wall, which collapses during inspiration.[11]

It is of key importance to perform a thorough preoperative evaluation given that nasal valve problems are often overlooked and the focus is placed only on the contributions from septal deviation and inferior turbinate hypertrophy. Inappropriate preoperative patient selection is closely associated with a patient's postoperative dissatisfaction.[4,5] Septoplasty has been shown to be effective for patients with obvious septal deviation. Long-term outcomes of septoplasty have been less successful for all categories of patients, however, when grouped together.[12] Jessen and colleagues[13] and Ho and colleagues[14] described redevelopment of nasal obstruction after septoplasty alone in as high as 50% of patients.

## Outcomes Studies of Functional Rhinoplasty

With the limitations of traditional septal and inferior turbinate surgery, surgeons have increasingly directed their attention to the nasal valve area. Indeed, it has been reported that patients with nasal valve collapse are plagued with a greater perception of nasal airway obstruction than those with septal deviation alone.[15] Functional rhinoplasty describes the collection of techniques that surgically addresses airflow by correcting nasal valve disturbances.

In recent years, a number of investigators have attempted to determine the efficacy of functional rhinoplasty techniques in addressing nasal obstruction. Rhee and colleagues[9] performed a 25-year systematic review of the literature searching for evidence supporting the role of functional rhinoplasty and nasal valve repair. He found substantial level IV evidence supporting the efficacy of modern day rhinoplasty techniques for treating nasal obstruction caused by nasal valve collapse.

The literature on functional rhinoplasty lacks randomized control trials, which are usually considered the gold standard and the highest levels of evidence in research. Given the ethical difficulties of blindly randomizing surgical procedures, it is not uncommon to rely on observational and retrospective studies to assess the impact of surgical treatments. Notably, the literature also lacks objective measurement tools to quantify nasal obstruction. Only 27% of the studies found in Rhee's and coworkers review had some type of objective assessment tool. These included validated quality-of-life surveys, such as the one used in the NOSE trial, whereas other studies used rhinomanometry or acoustic rhinometry whose clinical relevance have been questioned previously.[16,17] The NOSE scale, developed by Stewart and colleagues,[6] is one of the main validated evaluation instruments measuring subjective sensation of nasal obstruction and is one of the key accepted measures of postoperative success. Although this scale was initially used to evaluate septoplasty patients, it can be applied to different surgical procedures that address nasal obstruction.

Two studies have separated the effect of nasal valve correction from the septoplasty component. The combined septoplasty and nasal valve approach showed superior improvement in nasal obstruction over septoplasty alone.[12,18] Constantian and Brian[12] showed that internal and external valvular reconstruction increased airflow significantly, but the combination of nasal valve surgery in conjunction with septal surgery increased geometric mean airflow the most by almost five times.

Most[11] conducted a prospective study of 41 patients to measure the efficacy of functional rhinoplasty techniques with the validated NOSE questionnaire. Mean NOSE scores decreased in all patients who underwent functional rhinoplasty. There was a trend toward improved scores in patients who underwent turbinate reduction in conjunction with spreader grafting compared with those subjects who did not undergo these procedures.

The senior author was the principal investigator in the first multicenter, prospective study on quality of life following functional rhinoplasty. Preliminary data of 90 subjects who underwent nasal valve surgery by 12 surgeons across the United States indicate a clear quality-of-life improvement at 3, 6, and 12 months postoperatively as measured by the NOSE questionnaire. It is the hope of the senior author that this investigation and other studies will help to improve the state of third-party reimbursement for techniques used in functional rhinoplasty.

## ANATOMY

The external nasal valve refers to the distal most aperture of the nasal airway. Serving essentially as the nostril orifice, it consists primarily of fibrofatty tissues of the nasal alae in conjunction with the lower lateral cartilages (LLCs), columella, medial crural footplates, the caudal septum, and the piriform aperture.[5,19] The contribution of the external valve to nasal obstruction varies considerably depending on the individual anatomy of the nose (**Fig. 1**).

The internal nasal valve area describes the region of the nasal airway that typically corresponds to the area of greatest resistance to airflow. Pyramidal in shape, it functions as a choke point for nasal airflow and is comprised circumferentially by the caudal aspect of the ULC, the nasal septum, the head of the inferior turbinate, and piriform aperture and nasal floor. The internal valve area is of key importance because it is the critical area of resistance in the anterior nose, affecting nasal airflow by its dynamic regulation of the nasal airway cross-sectional area.[2,5] It is estimated that nasal valve dysfunction exists in approximately 13% of patients with nasal obstruction.[20] The internal nasal valve angle is the narrowest portion of the valve and usually measures 15 to 20 degrees in the leptorrhine nose. The average cross-sectional area of the internal nasal valve area is between 55 and 83 mm$^2$ (**Fig. 2**). There is some ambiguity in the literature regarding the exact anatomic landmarks that characterize the internal valve area. The previously mentioned description connotes it is a two-dimensional cross section at one point along the nasal airway. In reality, dynamic collapse in this region often occurs at the lateral wall of the nose posterior and caudal to the ULC and superoposterior to the lateral crura. This region between the internal valve area and external nasal valve, sometimes called the "intervalve" area, is typically deficient of nasal cartilage. Narrowing or weakness in this area is marked by noses with deep supra-alar creases and inspiratory lateral wall medialization. Narrow, projecting noses with a correspondingly narrow piriform aperture are more likely to demonstrate this abnormality (**Fig. 3**).

The nasal septum is a midline bony and cartilaginous structure that divides the nasal cavity in halves. Posterior and cephalad, the septum is comprised of bone: the perpendicular plate of the ethmoid and the vomer. Along its posterosuperior border, it is attached to the cribiform plate. At its cephalic border, the osseous septum attaches to the frontal bone and its posterior free edge forms the midline partition of the nasal choanae. Anteriorly and caudally, the septum is cartilaginous, formally termed the "quadrangular cartilage." Firm attachments to osseous structures cephalically (the osseous septum) and ventrally (the maxillary crest) form the basis of its stability. Anteriorly, the maxillary crest terminates at the nasal spine, the osseous attachment of the posterior septal angle of the quadrangular cartilage. Concavities and convexities of the nasal septum can narrow the airway and may compromise laminar airflow.

Dorsally and caudally, the cartilaginous septum is interconnected to the ULC and LLC, respectively. Dorsally, the paired, shield-like ULCs are fused in the midline to the dorsal edge of the cartilaginous septum. Caudally, the LLCs have an intimate relationship with the caudal edge of the septum. The inherent stiffness and thickness of the ULC and LLC contribute to the support of the nasal airway against inspiratory collapse.[5,19,21–24]

## PATHOPHYSIOLOGY

The nose serves a multitude of physiologic functions: immunologic, sensory, olfactory, and

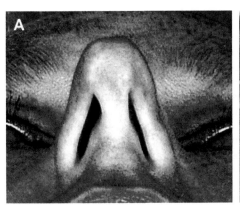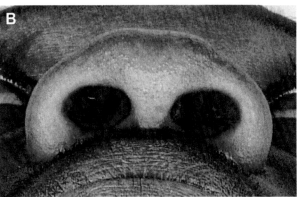

**Fig. 1.** (*A*) Narrow, projecting nose with external valve insufficiency. (*B*) Wide, flat nose with broadly patent external valves.

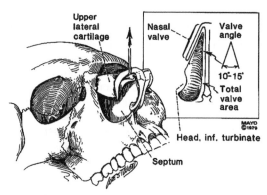

Fig. 2. The nasal valve area is bounded by nasal septum. Caudal end of upper lateral cartilage, and soft fibrofatty tissue overlying piriform aperture and floor of nose and posteriorly by the head of the inferior turbinate. This area is shaped like an inverted cone or teardrop, the slitlike apex of which is the nasal valve angle, and normally subtends an angle of 10 to 15 degrees. (*From* Kasperbauer JL, Kern EB. Nasal valve physiology. Otolaryngol Clin North Am 1987;20:792; with permission.)

respiratory. As a respiratory organ it performs a prominent regulatory role. Air enters the nasal cavity, where it is warmed to a temperature of approximately 31°C to 34°C, regardless of outside temperature. It also humidifies the inspired air to

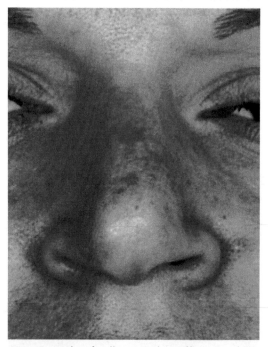

Fig. 3. Example of collapse and insufficiency of the lateral wall in the intervalve area. Patient has deep supra-alar creases, concave lateral crura, and inspiratory collapse.

a relative humidity of 90% to 95%.[2] These functions prevent desiccation of the distal airways, which allows optimal gas exchange, and helps maintain temperature homeostasis.

The physiologic role of the nasal valve is not as well defined. With forced inspiration by the nose, collapse of the valve occurs even in patients without nasal valve pathology. It is thought that nasal valve collapse dynamically regulates the cross-sectional area of the nasal cavity preventing the influx of excessive air and ensures proper warming, humidification, and filtration before entering the lungs. The regulation might also assist in olfaction. As the nasal valve narrows, turbulent airflow is created that is redirected toward the olfactory epithelium.[24]

The main factors that contribute to the airflow patterns are the nasal cavity geometry and the flow rate. As inspiration is initiated, airflow is directed in a laminar fashion toward the nasal valve region. This region has the smallest cross-sectional area and causes an acceleration of the flow. Poiseuille's law explains this phenomenon. This principle explains that the volume of a homogeneous fluid (air technically is a fluid) flowing through a tube per unit time (the definition of velocity) is directly proportional to the pressure difference between its ends and the fourth power of its internal radius. It is inversely proportional to the length of the tube and to the viscosity of the fluid. This equation predicts that even small changes in radius greatly affect the flow velocity by increasing it to the fourth power of the radius. Changes in pressure (essentially inspiratory effort) increase velocity, but not to the extent that does a change in radius.[25]

As flow velocity increases through constricted regions of the nasal airway, the Bernoulli theorem then predicts that air pressure decreases. This results in a negative pressure at the point of highest velocity, exerting a collapsing force on the surrounding tube. Whether or not this force leads to actual symptomatic collapse of the nasal airway depends on the magnitude of the force and the strength and geometry of the nasal valve areas. As described, the magnitude of the force depends on the pressure, which is determined by airflow velocity, which is determined by inspiratory effort and nasal airway dimension. The strength of the nasal airway depends on the anatomy of the nose, most notably the width and strength of the lateral nasal wall and the shape and stiffness of the ULC and LLC. The goals of functional rhinoplasty are twofold: to widen the nasal airway aperture and thereby reduce airflow velocity and the negative pressure created within the nose; and to strengthen the valve areas to become more resistant against collapsing pressure forces (**Fig. 4**).[26,27]

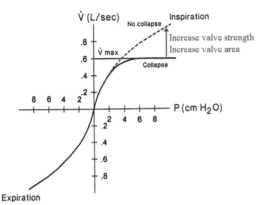

**Fig. 4.** Flow-volume curve demonstrating normal functioning nose (*dotted line*) and nose with valvular collapse (*solid line*). In the pathologic state, at high pressure (inspiratory effort) the nose collapses and no further increase in flow occurs. The goal of surgery is to widen and strengthen the airway in the nasal valve areas, and shift the flow-volume curve from abnormal to normal. (*From* Kasperbauer JL, Kern FB. Nasal valve physiology. Otolaryngol Clin North Am 1987;20:704; with permission.)

## ASSESSMENT

Nasal valve collapse occurs during dynamic inspiration. Examination and assessment of this area is difficult because the soft tissues easily become distorted and stretched with anterior rhinoscopy. In addition, physiologic collapse with deep inspiration can be seen in patients without nasal valve dysfunction. Inspection of the nasal valve without manipulation, such as with flexible nasopharyngocogopy, is valuable. Nasal valve dysfunction can be static, dynamic, or variable. In cases of static dysfunction, narrowing exists that is independent of air flow (eg, septal deviation or turbinate hypertrophy). Dynamic insufficiency is revealed only during active inspiration when poorly supported nasal valve structures collapse.

The Cottle maneuver is performed by placing lateral traction on the cheek to assist in nasal valve opening. The patient is then asked if they feel relief from their nasal obstruction. This assessment has low specificity and is not considered useful.[24] The modified Cottle maneuver is more effective in diagnosis. A fine instrument, such as a cerumen loop, is placed gently within the nares against the lateral nasal wall at the level of maximal observable collapse. The patient is then asked to breathe in through the nose. Collapse is stented by the instrument, which should be held lightly to prevent distortion. This maneuver may predict the potential benefit of surgical nasal valve correction.[28] The procedure should be performed both before and after decongestion to determine the effect of mucosal swelling in symptology.

A variety of objective tests have been used to measure nasal obstruction. Rhinomanometry and acoutic rhinometry are the most favored. A rhinomanometer measures nasal cavity pressure and flow and an acoustic rhinometer measures cross-sectional area and volume within the nasal cavity. Both instruments are used objectively to assess nasal patency. Studies regarding their validity are equivocal. Several articles show no correlation and others show only a moderate relationship between these techniques and a patient's subjective symptoms.[16,29,30] Following the trends in the literature, Kim and colleagues[16] found no significant correlation between rhinomanometry and acoustic rhinometry, and the severity of nasal airway obstruction. Overall, there is a need for a more objective measurement tools to evaluate nasal obstruction.

## SURGICAL TECHNIQUES
### Lateral Wall Insufficiency

No doubt because of the ambiguous anatomic terminology, the techniques (mostly structural cartilage grafts) used to correct lateral wall problems have not been classified consistently as either internal valve or external valve treatments. Furthermore, the actual locations of these grafts vary according to individual anatomy and pathophysiology; they cannot be consistently labeled as internal or external valve therapies. The authors view such a classification as overly simplistic and one that leads to confusion of a semantic nature. Instead, they view lateral wall reconstruction as a continuum of treatments that span from the internal valve area to the external valve. The graft techniques described in this section are discussed roughly from cephalad to caudal placement (although actual location of any of these grafts may be adjusted according to need).

### Alar batten grafts
Alar batten grafts are curved cartilaginous supports placed into areas of maximal lateral wall weakness, most typically posterior to the lateral crura. Through the external approach, the grafts are inserted into tight pockets that overlap and extend posterior to the lateral crura. The curvature of the graft is oriented to lateralize the supra-alar area (**Fig. 5**). The lateral aspect of the graft may be caudal to or cephalad to the lateral crura depending on the area of maximal pinching. The grafts may extend beyond the pyriform aperture to add maximal support. In cases in which lateral recurvature of the native lateral crura impinges on the nostril width, the lateral crura may be sutured to the alar batten grafts for lateral stabilization. Internal

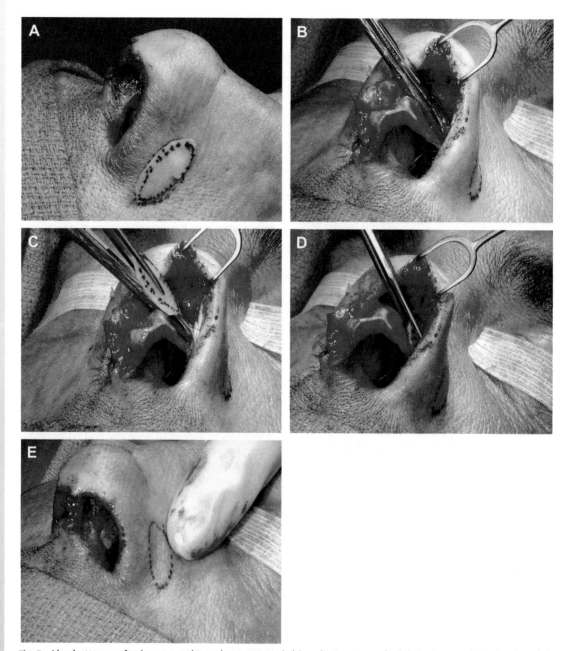

**Fig. 5.** Alar batten graft placement through an external rhinoplasty approach. (*A*) An appropriate-sized graft is carved and placed superficially over the marked optimal position. (*B*) A precise pocket is dissected from the posterior termination of the lateral crus to a point over the piriform aperture. (*C*) The graft is placed snugly within the pocket. (*D*) The graft should extend to or beyond the piriform aperture. (*E*) After graft placement, palpation confirms correct placement.

vestibular stents may be placed in the postoperative period to prevent postoperative medialization of the lateral wall. These stents may be constructed with pliable plastic stents or sections of nasal-pharyngeal tubes[31] and may be maintained in the nasal vestibules while the patient sleeps for a period of months following surgery (**Fig. 6**).

The size of the alar batten graft may vary depending on the severity of obstruction to be treated. In general, the longer, wider, and more curved the graft, the greater effect it has on supporting and widening the lateral wall. In some cases, septal cartilage possesses some inherent curvature making it suitable for an alar batten graft.

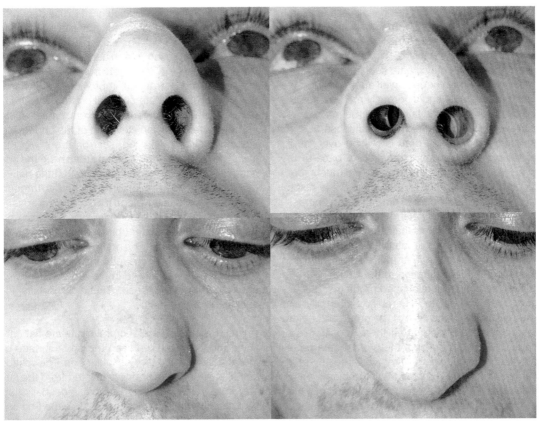

**Fig. 6.** Splints can be used intranasally to support lateralized healing of alar batten grafts. Cylindric sections of nasopharyngeal tubes may serve as effective splints.

If significant curvature is desired, conchal cartilage may be more suitable. In the most severe of cases, alar batten grafts may be fashioned to be quite long, spanning from the mid-portion of the lateral crus to a point lateral to the lip of the piriform aperture. Such grafts, however, are more likely to create palpable and visible distortion to the external nose.

Through open rhinoplasty, it is important to place the graft within a precise pocket that corresponds to the area of maximal pinching or narrowing as determined preoperatively with the modified Cottle maneuver. Rather than being placed in one consistent anatomic position, the optimal location for alar batten grafts varies from patient to patient. For example, with cephalically malpositioned lateral crura, it is more likely that there is a deficiency of support caudal to the lateral crura. In other cases in which there is poor support of the supra-alar lateral wall, the grafts may be placed cephalad to the lateral crura. The submuscular pocket should be dissected accurately to match the dimensions of the graft so that mobility of the graft is minimized. Should an overly large pocket

be made inadvertently, the graft may be fixated to surrounding tissue with fine absorbable sutures.

An endonasal approach may also be used to place alar batten grafts. In this technique, a marginal incision is made and scissor dissection is executed over the surface of the lateral crura toward the desired pocket for the graft. In most situations this requires that the vector of dissection start superolaterally to establish the plane immediately superficial to the lateral crus, then the dissection redirected in a true lateral (posterior) direction toward the lateral wall and piriform aperture. If this direction change does not occur and the pocket is made too high (cephalad), an unsightly bulge may ensue above the alar crease with no significant improvement in lateral wall support. Once the correct snug pocket is made, the graft may be inserted through the marginal incision into the desired location and orientation.

In some situations, the alar batten graft may cause an undesired contour bulge internally in the nose along the alar sidewall. In some cases, this may lead to exacerbation of the airway obstruction rather than correction. Three scenarios in which this may occur are discussed. First, the problem may be caused by malposition of the graft such that it slips medial to the lip of the piriform aperture and collapses inward. A short graft or a short dissected pocket may create such a problem. This problem may even happen well after surgery if the patient repeatedly and vigorously manipulates the inside of the nose and lateral wall. Second, a very narrow piriform aperture may predispose to such problems, even if the graft is resting over the lip of the bone. Essentially, the skeletal base of the nose is so narrow that there is not much room for a lateral wall graft. In such cases, it is helpful to use an outwardly curved graft that can compensate for the relatively narrow airway geometry. Third, other techniques that narrow or medialize the domes may pull the lateral termination of the lateral crura medially. This mass effect may lead to inward, medial migration of the lateral crura.

To avoid the aforementioned problems, the surgeon must inspect the lateral wall internally and externally after placement of the grafts and before the completion of surgery. If there is evidence of undesired inward bulging, the graft should be repositioned or modified. Often, a larger or more curved graft can overcome these problems. Alternatively, the alar batten graft may be replaced with an extended lateral crural strut (discussed next). In equivocal cases, the lateral wall and alar batten graft may be supported during the postoperative period with either internal splints or full-thickness lateral wall bolsters, both of which may aid in maintaining optimal graft position. In some cases, patients are advised to use internal stents intermittently over the first 6 to 12 months (period of maximal soft tissue contracture) to promote long-term healing of the grafts in favorable position.

### Lateral crural struts and lateral crural grafts

In most noses, the native lateral crura impart a fair amount of support to the nasal tip and lateral wall. In some noses, however, inherent weakness, cephalic malposition, or iatrogenic injury of the lateral crura leads to reduced support in these areas. This is particularly true when the overall geometry of the nose is projecting, narrow, and thin. Such noses are characterized by narrow piriform apertures, thin alar side walls, and concave alar margins. In these cases, structural reinforcement of the native lateral crura may be indicated. Two types of grafts are commonly used to achieve this end.

The lateral crural strut is an underlay graft placed between the vestibular lining and undersurface of the lateral crus. The lateral crural graft is an overlay graft placed superficial to the lateral crus. In both cases, the grafts can add to the strength and support of weak or compromised native cartilages. Selection of which graft to use depends on several factors, cosmetic considerations included among them. For example, lateral crural grafts are often used in conjunction with a shield graft to soften the transition from the tip to the alar lobule and lateral wall, improving overall nasal base triangularity. Lateral crural grafts are also favored when the native lateral crura are severely compromised or when elevation of the underlying vestibular skin is risky (eg, scar or atrophy of the lining). In contrast, lateral crural struts have the advantage of being a hidden graft, so that the native cartilage continues to impart the contour through the skin soft tissue envelope (SSTE). This is advantageous in a thin-skinned individual, in whom an onlay graft has a greater chance to transmit an irregularity. Both types of grafts may be used to stiffen and straighten the lateral crura to reinforce a weak lateral wall and to improve triangularity to a misshapen nasal base. Technical details for each type of graft follow.

**Lateral crural strut**  Lateral crural struts are flat cartilage grafts placed between the undersurface of the lateral crura and the vestibular skin. The vestibular skin should be carefully elevated from the lateral crura from cephalad to caudal. A cephalic trim is generally required to gain access to the free cephalic edge of the lateral crura to execute this dissection. The amount of cartilage removed during the cephalic trim varies depending on the need for volume reduction, but in most cases (because the lateral crural strut technique leads to some flattening of the lateral crura) minimal excision is needed. The caudal attachment of the lateral crus and skin should remain intact to prevent caudal migration of the graft.

Once the epithelium is elevated, the graft should be positioned at the undersurface of the lateral crura to extend from just lateral to the domes to the lateral aspect of the lateral crura or just beyond. The lateral crural strut graft should be secured to the LLC with two to three horizontal mattress 5.0 clear nylon or PDS sutures. The underlying vestibular mucosa should then be apposed to the undersurface of the lateral crural struts with full-thickness chromic suture. Because these grafts need to be thin, straight (or very slightly convex outward), and strong, septal cartilage is ideally suited as a source material. Rib cartilage is also an effective donor source, although the carving of the graft from rib is more difficult (should result in no more than 1 mm thick, but fairly straight graft). Because of its curvature and softness, ear cartilage makes poor material for these grafts. The overall dimensions of the lateral crural strut varies but may range from 2 to 3 cm in length,

6 to 10 mm in width, and about 1 mm in width (**Fig. 7**).

The lateral crural strut has two main effects. First, it stiffens the lateral crura, allowing it to provide more support to the lateral wall and tip of the nose. Second, it allows for straightening of a convex, concave, or distorted lateral crus. By virtue of the graft's inherent stiffness and shape, the mattress sutures between the lateral crura and the strut graft force the lateral crura into a straighter orientation. This effect may be enhanced when an intradomal suture is combined with the lateral crural graft (a common combination used to refine cosmetically a strong cartilage bulbous tip). In some noses, the lateral crura are fairly straight except for the lateral termination of the cartilage, which recurves inward, much like medial crural footplates may curve laterally. Placing a lateral crural strut that extends just beyond the tail of the lateral crura is an effective way to treat such a problem. From an airway perspective, the stiffening and straightening effects of the lateral crural strut may have a profound impact in adding strength to the lateral wall of the nose, reducing inspiratory collapse.

The extended lateral crural strut with repositioning of the lateral crura is a powerful variation of the strut technique. In this method, the native lateral crura are completely dissected free from the underlying vestibular epithelial bed and left connected to the intermediate crura at the domes. A longer strut graft is sutured to the undersurface of the lateral crus, starting at the desired dome position and extending up to 1.5 cm beyond the termination of the tail of the lateral crus. This extended portion of the lateral crural strut is placed into a precise pocket overhanging the piriform aperture, much like the pocket created for the alar batten graft. The caudal-cephalic position of the pocket depends on desired graft and lateral crural position, but is generally placed quite caudal along the lateral wall. This allows for caudal repositioning of cephalically malpositioned lateral crura. This allows for strengthening of the nose from tip to alar base, making this technique very useful for noses with severe collapse globally along the lateral wall. This technique may also be used to improve triangularity to the tip and base of the nose. Precise and symmetric placement of the pockets and creation of

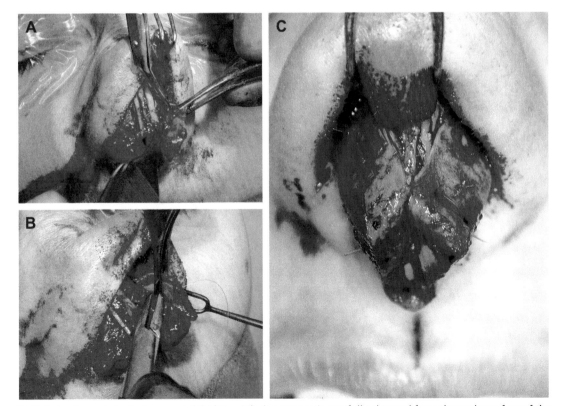

**Fig. 7.** Lateral crural strut placement. (*A*) The vestibular mucosa is carefully elevated from the undersurface of the lateral crus. (*B*) The stiff lateral crural strut is sutured to the undersurface of the lateral crus. (*C*) The lateral crural struts should have the effect of stiffening and straightening the lateral crura. This supports the lateral wall against collapse and can improve triangularity to the base and tip of the nose.

these grafts is critical to create a symmetric nose with appropriate tip position and shape (**Fig. 8**).

Patients who undergo lateral crural struts should understand that there is noticeable contour edge along the internal aspect of the vestibule and lateral wall. This may lead to a slight obstruction of mucous egress in the nose in some patients, but with proper hygiene typically does not lead to a problem.

**Lateral crural graft** Lateral crural grafts may serve many of the same functions as the lateral crural

strut. As discussed previously, these grafts are placed on the superficial surface of the lateral crura instead of the undersurface. Like the lateral crural strut, the lateral crural graft can provide support, stiffening, and straightening of the native lateral crura. The shape, length, and orientation may also be modulated to fit the need of the given patient. The main difficulty with the lateral crural graft is the contribution to external contour. Because it sits superficial to the lateral crura, the graft directly transmits through the skin envelope. This may be acceptable for an individual with thick skin but

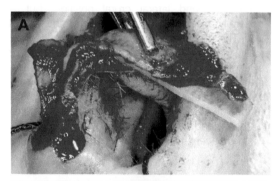

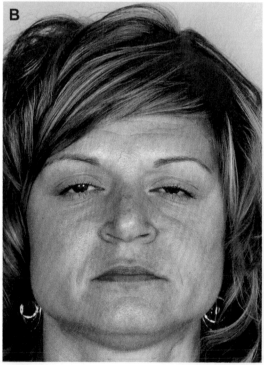

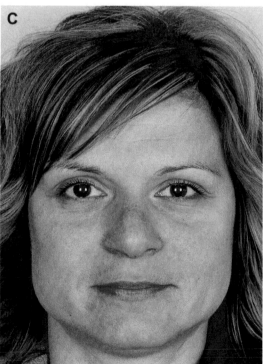

**Fig. 8.** An extended lateral crural strut with caudal repositioning of the lateral crura achieves both functional and aesthetic enhancement of the lateral wall and base of the nose. (*A*) The lateral crus is dissected completely free from the subjacent epithelium and a lateral crural strut, which extends beyond the termination of the lateral crus, is sutured to the undersurface. The extension of the graft is placed into a precise posterolateral pocket. Preoperative (*B, D, F*) and postoperative (*C, E, G*) views of patient who underwent this technique to correct functional and cosmetic problems related to concave, cephalically malpositioned lateral crura.

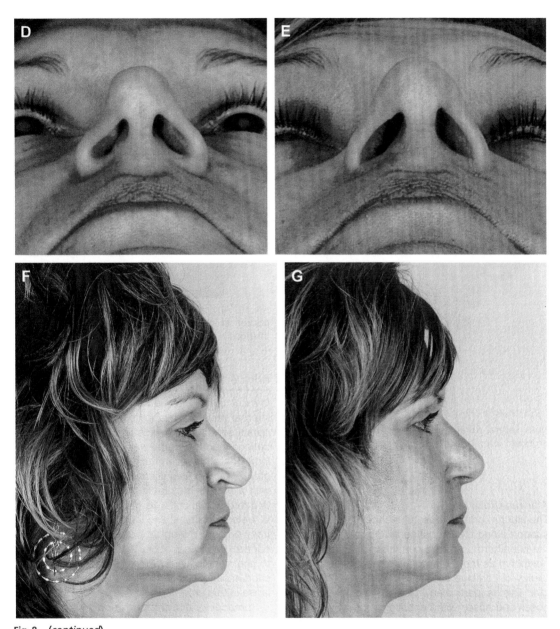

**Fig. 8.** (*continued*).

may lead to visible deformities in the thin skin nose.

The lateral crural graft may be useful in revision rhinoplasty when the native lateral crura are missing or are so damaged that they do not provide enough substrate for the lateral crural strut method. In these cases, the grafts may also be termed "lateral crural replacement grafts." Adequate stiffness, length, and strength of the graft are needed to overcome the lateral wall weakness and collapse in these cases. Precise contouring of the graft with smooth beveled edges is necessary

to create appropriate external form. The graft may be suture stabilized medially to whatever LLC remnant is available. Along its length, the graft should be sutured to the underlying scar and soft tissue bed (and cartilage remnants if available). Laterally, the graft may either be secured into a pocket over the piriform aperture or sutured to the dense fibrous deep alar tissue. In some cases, the lateral crural grafts may also be used to support and camouflage the leading anterior edge of a shield tip graft, which extends above the native domes (**Fig. 9**).

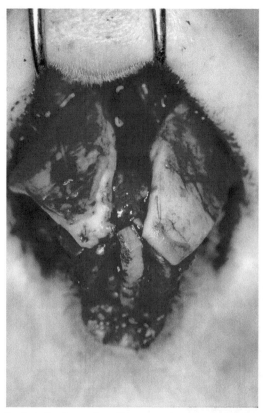

Fig. 9. Lateral crural graft to reconstruct severely compromised lateral crura.

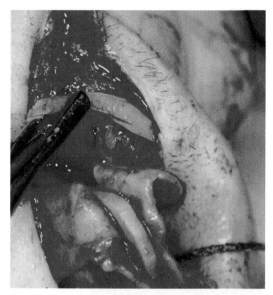

Fig. 10. Alar rim graft being inserted into precise pocket at the alar margin through the marginal incision.

### Alar rim grafts

The alar rim graft is a useful technique to provide support along the caudal nostril margin. Because the lateral crura diverge cephalad away from the nostril rim as they extend laterally, there is a deficiency of cartilage support along the nostril margin. This is particularly true in thin, projecting noses and noses with cephalic malpostion of the lateral crura. The alar rim graft adds cartilage support in this area of structural deficiency. These long, narrow cartilaginous grafts are placed into precise pockets along the alar rim just caudal to the marginal incision. They measure 1 to 3 mm in thickness and width and 5 to 8 mm in length. The medial aspect of these grafts may be gently bruised to aid in camouflage. They may be stabilized to the surrounding soft tissue or to the lateral aspect of the domal cartilages or a shield graft with a fine absorbable suture. These grafts provide modest support against caudal lateral wall insufficiency. They also improve the concave or pinched appearance of the rim on base view and create a more triangular appearance to the tip and base of the nose (**Fig. 10**).

### Middle Vault Insufficiency

In most cases, the middle vault, the ULCs, and the internal valve proper (angle between the ULC and dorsal septum) have less functional airway implications than the lateral wall of the nose. In certain individuals, however, the middle vault can take on greater airway significance. Specifically, noses with a narrow middle vault, a projecting dorsum, or inferomedial collapse of the ULC and inverted-V deformity (typically iatrogenic complications from primary rhinoplasty cartilaginous dorsal reduction) are susceptible to obstruction referable to the middle vault. In particular, patients with short nasal bones and long ULCs are at risk of collapse in this area.

Spreader grafts are long rectangular cartilaginous grafts placed between the dorsal cartilaginous septum and ULC. These grafts are useful to correct functional and cosmetic problems related to a narrow or asymmetric middle vault. These grafts are also used in primary rhinoplasty to prevent ULC collapse in high-risk patients. In particular, when reduction of a cartilaginous dorsal hump leads to excision of the horizontal articulation of the dorsal septum and ULCs, spreader grafts stabilize the middle vault and help restore appropriate horizontal width.

The dimensions of spreader grafts vary depending on specific needs and anatomy, but range from 6 to 12 mm in length, 3 to 5 mm in height, and 2 to 4 mm in thickness. More than one graft may be needed depending on available grafting material and the deformities. In general, the thicker aspect of the spreader graft is beveled and then positioned cephalad at the rhinion to create the normal appearance of slightly increased width in this area. The grafts may be placed from a dorsal approach after the ULCs are freed from the septum. Mucoperichondrial flaps must first be elevated from the junction of the ULC and septum to prevent injury to the mucosal lining and subsequent cicatrix. Two 5.0 PDS mattress sutures placed through the ULC, spreaders, and septum should be used for stabilization. The caudal ULC should be pulled caudally during the suture stabilization to straighten any redundancy or curvature. The dorsal profile of the spreader grafts, ULC, and septum should be coplanar and smooth. In situ trimming of the grafts may be needed to ensure an even dorsal surface (**Fig. 11**).

An alternative method of placement of spreader grafts is through a tight subperichondrial tunnel at

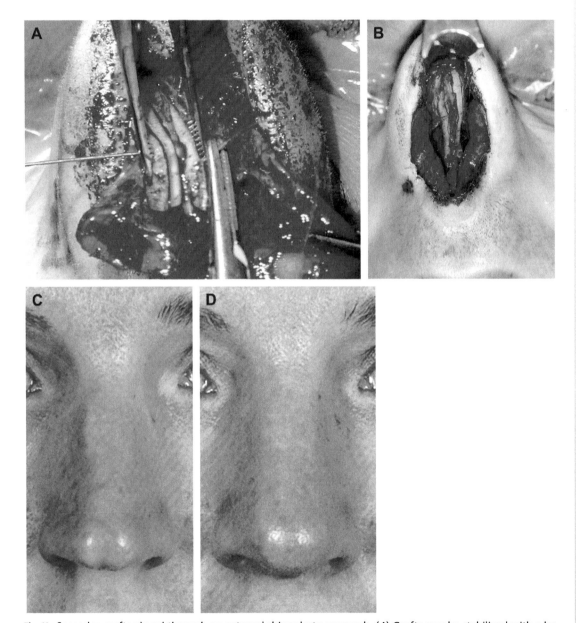

**Fig. 11.** Spreader grafts placed through an external rhinoplasty approach. (*A*) Grafts may be stabilized with a hypodermic needle to facilitate suture placement. (*B*) Appearance of spreader grafts between the dorsal margin of the septal cartilage and upper lateral cartilages. (*C*) Preoperative view of patient with pinched middle vault. (*D*) Postoperative view after spreader grafts.

the junction of the ULC and dorsal septum. In this method, elevation of the septal flaps must not include the dorsal aspect of the quadrilateral cartilage. A mucoperichondrial incision is made high on the septum just caudal to the junction of the ULC and septum. A narrow dissection instrument, such as a Freer elevator, is then used to create a long tight pocket just beneath the dorsal junction between the ULC and septum. Snug placement of a spreader graft into this tunnel cantilevers the ULC away from the dorsal septum, effecting additional widening of the internal nasal valve, as compared with placement of spreaders through an open dorsal approach. In the latter, the ULC is lateralized, but the absolute angle between the septum and ULC does not change. The precise pocket spreader graft creates lateralization and mild flaring of the ULC, leading to increased width and angulation. This effect is achieved because of the bulk of the spreader graft placed below the intact connection between the dorsal margin of the septum and the ULC. This translates to additional airway improvement. This method should be considered in patients with severe obstruction referable to the internal valve. A drawback to this method is the additional width that is incurred. Careful patient selection is required.[32,33]

### Brief Comments about Septal Surgery

The nasal septum represents the most common offending structure causing nasal obstruction. Traditional septal surgery is widely performed and is discussed quite extensively in the literature. Modification of the nasoseptal L strut is less commonly performed, but may be the aspect of the nasal septum creating obstruction. Dorsal deviations may contribute to internal valve area insufficiency and caudal septal deflections may impinge on the external nasal valve. Both dorsal and caudal septal deformities may lead to a crooked nose. Although not reviewed in detail in this manuscript, septal surgery is a critical aspect of the treatment of nasal obstruction in general and nasal valve problems in particular. Because of space limitations the interested reader is referred to other sources detailing the technical aspects of septal surgery.

## ALTERNATE SURGICAL TECHNIQUES

Alar batten and spreader grafts have often been referred to as the "workhorses" of functional rhinoplasty surgery. A wide array of techniques has been described in the literature, however, for the correction of nasal valve stenosis or collapse. Most of these alternate methods have not become universally accepted, primarily because they tend to address only one factor in what is usually a multifactorial problem. In addition, much of the literature supporting these techniques are limited to subjective outcomes measures. Although the techniques previously mentioned are the preferred techniques used by the authors, the following methods may be valuable in certain instances for particular patient problems. A brief description of some notable examples of these techniques follows.

### Butterfly Graft

The butterfly graft is essentially a structurally supportive onlay graft that is placed across the nasal dorsum in the vicinity of the internal valve area. Typically constructed with the entirety of one ear's conchal cartilage, the graft is configured into a symmetric "v" shape with its tip pointing caudally. Essentially, the lateral "wings" of the butterfly graft are pushed downward on the ULCs as they are sutured in place to create outward tension. The cephalic edge of the graft is positioned superior to the caudal edges of the ULCs so that it confers an outward spring effect to widen the middle vault (similar mechanics as flaring sutures). The caudal edge of the graft is deep to the cephalic edge of the LLCs to minimize external contour distortion. The middle vault dorsum can be lowered slightly before placement of the graft to accommodate the thickness of the graft while preserving the pre-existing dorsal height and contour. The graft is then secured with several 5.0 PDS sutures. Clark and Cook[34] studied this technique as it applied to revision rhinoplasty patients, and found that 97% reported complete resolution of their nasal airway obstruction (total N = 72). Eighty-six percent of patients reported an improvement in their cosmetic appearance and those that perceived unsatisfactory cosmetic results stated they would have undergone the surgery again to obtain the nasal patency benefits.

### Flaring Sutures

This technique uses a horizontal mattress suture placed between the two ULCs, using the nasal dorsum as a fulcrum. By means of an open approach to nose the caudal and lateral aspect of the ULC is exposed. A 5.0 clear nylon horizontal mattress stitch is placed in the mid-portion of each ULC, traversing over the cartilaginous bridge of the nose. As the stitch is tightened, the ULCs flare outward, which increases the nasal valve angle. Schlosser and Park[19] described the use of flaring sutures aimed at increasing the internal nasal valve angle in cadaver studies. A total of 34 cadavers underwent this procedure and then acoustic rhinometry and rhinomanometry where used to measure mean cross-sectional area and airway patency. They found that flaring sutures and spreader grafts, in combination, significantly increased cross-sectional area by 18.7%, with a statistically significant increase in nasal patency. Each procedure individually did not significantly increase mean cross-sectional area and spreader grafts showed the least amount of increase overall. Critics of this technique point out that there is likely to be a relaxation of the suture effect on the framework of the nose over time. In addition, there may be risk of a "cheese-string" migration of the suture through the cartilage, causing relaxation of the initial tension created.

## Suture Suspension Techniques

These methods focus on widening the lateral wall of the nose by fixating the lateral crura to lateral anchor point. Menger[35] describes a lateral crural tuck-up technique in which a delivery approach is used to access the lateral aspect of the lateral crura. A drill hole is then made at the piriform aperture and a strong permanent suture is used to fixate the lateral crus to the bony pyramid. As the suture is tightened the lateral crus flares outward in a superolateral direction, widening the angle formed by the lateral nasal wall. Menger described a series of seven patients most of whom reported improved subjective normal nasal breathing and on forced inspiration as compared with before surgery at 3, 6, and 9 months postoperatively. Variations on this technique include using an orbital rim anchor point[36,37] or using a bone anchor suspension technique.[38] Concerns regarding the long-term relaxation of suture-derived tensioning of tissue have been raised regarding these techniques.

## Alloplastic Valve Implants

Mendelson and Golchin[39] described the placement of high-density porus polyethylene implants for the prevention of dynamic collapse. These alloplastic implants, fashioned into the shape of batten grafts, were sutured directly onto the lateral crura in conjunction with suture suspension. The implants were intended to provide structural stabilization and to prevent the sutures from pulling through. In their series, Mendelson and Golchin[39] reviewed 40 patients and found that 92% of them experienced "good" improvement in their nasal airway (subjective patient evaluation). Improvement in nasal airway patency (as measured by physical examination) was statistically significant. Although widening of the lower third of the nose was noticeable in some cases, cosmetic outcome was satisfactory, with 42% of patients rating their appearance as better than preoperatively and 52% indicating they did not see a difference in their appearance. In recent years, other alloplastic products have become available as an option for lateral wall supportive grafting. To date, there is a lack of long-term data available regarding the safety and efficacy of such implants.

## Nasal Valve Dilators

Multiple devices are available on the market designed to increase nasal valve patency. These products target people with snoring difficulties or athletes. Adhesive external nasal dilator strips are applied to the skin of the nose by gently folding the strip so that it contours the external nasal shape at the level of the nasal valve. Flexible polyester springs exist within the strip, which recoil backward from the bent position. Because the strip is firmly adherent to the skin, the recoil generates a superolateral force on the external nasal valve causing it to open. These devices were found to dilate the nasal airway significantly by reducing resistance, but also helped stiffen the lateral nasal wall preventing inspiratory collapse.[40,41] Roithmann and Chapnik[42] found that 33 patients with nasal obstruction, compared with 51 healthy controls, had significant increase in airway patency with the adhesive nasal strip, as measured by rhinomanometry and acoustic rhinometry. All subjects showed objective measures of increased patency and, except those with mucosal swelling, experienced subjective improvement in sensation of airflow.[42] Racial differences in basic nasal features explain findings that platyrrhine noses often respond paradoxically with an increase in resistance, and overall African Americans seem to have no significant change in nasal resistance when applying nasal valve dilators.[43,44] Another available product is the Nozovent nasal alar dilator. This consists of a semicircle of plastic with flattened free edges. The semicircle is squeezed and introduced into the nasal cavity with the flat free edges lying against nasal vestibule mucosa at the level of the nasal valve. As the plastic ring is released it recoils outward, exerting a lateral force on the internal nasal valve, expanding it. Although it is not as well tolerated, increased nasal patency and decreased resistance similar to (and occasionally better than) the external adhesive strips have been found.[44,45]

## SUMMARY

Obstruction at the level of the internal and external nasal valves is often an integral part of severe nasal obstruction but is frequently overlooked. One must address these areas surgically to improve nasal airflow dynamics maximally and alleviate the patient's perception of obstructed nasal breathing.

## REFERENCES

1. Couch ME, Blaugrund J, Kunar D, et al. Physical examination, and the preoperative evaluation. In: Cummings CW, editor. Otolaryngology head and neck surgery. Pennsylvania: Mosby; 1998. p. 3–25.
2. Behrbohm H. The dual character of nasal surgery. In: Behrbohm H, Tardy ME Jr, editors. Essentials of septorhinoplasty. Stuttgard Germany: Thieme; 2004. p. 2–7.
3. Toriumi DM, Josen J, Weinberger M, et al. Use of alar batten grafts for correction of nasal valve collapse. Arch Otolaryngol Head Neck Surg 1997;123(8):802–8.
4. Borges Dinis P, Haider H. Septoplasty: long-term evaluation of results. Am J Otolaryngol 2002;23:85–90.
5. Haight JSF, Cole P. The site and function of the nasal valve. Laryngoscope 1983;93:49–55.
6. Stewart MG, Smith TL, Weaver EM, et al. Outcomes after nasal septoplasty: results from the Nasal Obstruction Septoplasty Effectiveness (NOSE) Study. Am J Otolaryngol 2004;130:283–90.
7. Sedwick JD, Lopez AB, Gajewski BJ, et al. Caudal septoplasty for treatment of septal deviation: aesthetic and functional correction of the nasal base. Arch Facial Plastic Surg 2005;7:158–62.
8. Most SP. Anterior septal reconstruction: outcomes after a modified extracorporeal septoplasty technique. Arch Facial Plast Surg 2006;8:202–7.
9. Rhee JS, Arganbright JM, Mcmullin BT, et al. Evidence supporting functional rhinoplasty or nasal valve repair: a 25-year systematic review. Otolaryngol Head Neck Surg 2008;139:10–20.
10. Singh A, Patel N, Kenyon G, et al. Is there objective evidence that septal surgery improves nasal airflow? J Layrngol Otol 2006;120:916–20.
11. Most SP. Analysis of outcomes after functional rhinoplasty using a disease-specific quality of life instrument. Arch Facial Plast Surg 2006;8:306–9.
12. Constantian MB, Brian CR. The relative importance of septal and nasal valvular surgery in correcting airway obstruction in primary and secondary rhinoplasty. Plast Reconstr Surg 1996;98:38–54.
13. Jessen M, Ivarsson A, Malm L. Nasal airway resistance and symptoms after functional septoplasty: comparison of findings at 9 months and 9 years. Clin Otolaryngol Allied Sci 1989;14:231–4.
14. Ho WK, Yuen AP, Tang KC, et al. Time course in the relief of nasal blockage after septal and turbinate surgery: a prospective study. Arch Otolaryngol Head Neck Surg 2004;130:324–8.
15. Rhee JS, Book DT, Burzynski M, et al. Quality of life assessment in nasal airway obstruction. Laryngoscope 2003;113:1118–22.
16. Kim CS, Moon BK, Jung DH, et al. Correlation between nasal obstruction symptoms and objective parameters of acoustic rhinometry and rhinomanometry. Auris Nasus Larynx 1998;25:45–8.
17. Zambetti G, Filiaci F, Romeo R, et al. Assessment of cottle's areas through the application of a mathematical model deriving from acoustic rhinometry and rhinomanometric data. Clin Otolaryngol 2005;30:128–34.
18. Ricci E, Palonta F, Preti G, et al. Role of nasal valve in the surgically corrected nasal respiratory obstruction: evaluation through rhinomanometry. Am J Rhinol 2001;15:307–10.
19. Schlosser RJ, Park SS. Surgery for the dysfunctional nasal valve: cadaveric analysis and clinical outcomes. Arch Facial Plast Surg 1999;1(2):105–10.
20. Elwany S, Thabet H. Obstruction of the nasal valve. J Laryngol Otol 1996;100:221–4.
21. Ballenger JJ. The clinical anatomy and physiology of the nose and accessory sinuses. In: Ballenger JJ, editor. Diseases of the nose, throat, and ear. 12th edition. Philadelphia: Lea & Febiger; 1977. p. 1–22.
22. Jafek BW, Dodson BT, et al. Nasal obstruction. In: Bailey BJ, editor. Head and neck surgery—otolaryngology. 2nd edition. Philadelphia: Lippincott-Raven; 1998. p. 371–7.
23. Tardy ME, Brown RJ. Surgical anatomy of the nose. New York: Lippincott-Raven; 1990. p. 1–98.
24. Dolan RW. Nasal valve and nasal alar dysfunction. Facial Plast Surg Clin North Am 2000;8:447–64.
25. Sutera SP, Skalak R. The history of Poiseuille's law. Annu Rev Fluid Mech 1993;25:1–19.
26. Kelly JT, Prasad AK, Wexler AS. Detailed flow patterns in the nasal cavity. J Appl Physiol 2000;89:323–37.
27. Wen J, Inthavong K, Tu J, et al. Numerical simulations for the detailed airflow dynamics in a human nasal cavity. Respir Physiol Neurobiol 2008;161:125–35.
28. Constantinides MS, Adamson PA, Cole P. The long-term effects of open cosmetic septorhinoplasty on nasal air flow. Arch Otolaryngol Head Neck Surg 1996;122(1):41–5.
29. Warren DW, Hairfield WM, Seaton DL. The relationship between nasal airway cross-sectional area and nasal resistance. Am J Orthod Dentofac Orthop 1987;92:390–5.
30. Naito K, Cole P, Chaban R, et al. Nasal resistance, sensation of obstruction and rhinoscopic findings compared. Am J Rhinol 1988;2:65–9.
31. Egan KK, Kim DW. A novel intranasal stent for functional rhinoplasty and nostril stenosis. Laryngoscope 2005;115:903–9.
32. Fischer H, Gubisch W. Nasal valves–importance and surgical procedures. Facial Plast Surg 2006;22:266–80.
33. Ballert JA, Park SS. Functional rhinoplasty: treatment of the dysfunctional nasal sidewall. Plast Surg 2006;22:49–54.

34. Clark JM, Cook TA. The butterfly graft in functional secondary rhinoplasty. Laryngoscope 2002;112:1917–25.

35. Menger DJ. Lateral crus pull-up: a method for collapse of the external nasal valve. Arch Facial Plast Surg 2006;8:333–7.

36. Paniello RC. Nasal valve suspension: an effective treatment for nasal valve collapse. Arch Otolaryngol Head Neck Surg 1996;122:1342–6.

37. Lee DS, Glasgold AI. Correction of nasal valve stenosis with lateral suture suspension. Arch Facial Plast Surg 2001;3:237–40.

38. Friedman M, Ibrahim H, Lee G, et al. A simplified techniques for airway correction at the nasal valve area. Otol Head Neck Surg 2004;131:519–24.

39. Mendelson MS, Golchin K. Alar expansion and reinforcement: a new technique to manage nasal valve collapse. Arch Facial Plast Surg 2006;8:293–9.

40. Kirkness JP, Wheatley JR, Amis TC. Nasal airflow dynamics: mechanisms and responses associated with an external nasal dilator strip. Eur Respir J 2000;15:929–36.

41. Peltonen LI, Vento SI, Simola M, et al. Effects of the nasal strip and dilator on nasal breathing: a study with healthy subjects. Rhinology 2004;42:122–5.

42. Roithmann R, Chapnik J. Role of the external nasal dilator in the management of nasal obstruction. Laryngoscope 1998;108:712–5.

43. Portugal LG, Mehta RH, Smith BE, et al. Objective assessment of the breathe-right device during exercise in adult males. Am J Rhinol 1997;11:393–7.

44. Ellegard E. Mechanical nasal alar dilators. Rhinol 2006;44:239–48.

45. Petruson B. Snoring can be reduced when the nasal airflow is increased by the nasal dilator nozovent. Arch Otol Head Neck Surg 1990;116:462–4.

# Cleft Lip Rhinoplasty

Jonathan M. Sykes, MD, FACS[a],*, Yong Ju. Jang, MD[b]

**KEYWORDS**

• Diagnosis • Management • Cleft lip nasal deformity

The cleft nasal deformity associated with congenital cleft lip malformations presents a formidable challenge for any facial plastic surgeon. The extent of the nasal deformity may range from mild to severe, and is related to the extent of the original lip abnormality.[1] A nasal deformity is associated with all cleft lip deformities, which is evidenced by the nasal tip and alar base asymmetry found in patients with mild microform clefting of the lip.

The cleft nasal deformity is a three-dimensional abnormality involving all layers of the nose, beginning with the skeletal platform and extending into the vestibular lining, cartilaginous infrastructure, and external nasal skin.[2] The fact that cleft noses have abnormalities in all tissue layers separates them in kind and difficulty from most cosmetic rhinoplasties.

The nasal abnormalities associated with congenital cleft lips are characteristic, varying only by the extent of the original deformity and by whether the clefting of the lip is unilateral or bilateral. The secondary cleft nasal deformity, however, is more variable. It relates to three factors:

> The original congenital malformation
> Any repositioning and surgical scarring resulting from prior surgical intervention
> Alterations of the nose related to growth

Many surgical approaches and techniques have been described to repair cleft nasal deformities. Because the presenting patient with a congenital deformity is young, the surgical plan must account for patient growth and surgical scarring. The surgeon should understand the pathophysiology of the deformity and have a systematic surgical plan. This article describes the classic nasal abnormalities associated with clefting of the lip, and outlines surgical techniques and timing used to minimize these deformities.

## ANATOMY OF THE CLEFT NASAL DEFORMITY
### Unilateral Cleft Nasal Deformity

The nasal deformities associated with congenital unilateral cleft lips have been well described and are consistent.[3,4] The extent of the typical nasal deformity is related to the degree of deficiency of alar base support on the cleft side. The typical characteristics of the unilateral cleft lip nose are described in **Box 1**.

The hallmark of the unilateral cleft lip nasal deformity is a three-dimensional asymmetry of the nasal tip and alar base (**Fig. 1**). The columella and caudal nasal septum always deviate to the noncleft side, secondary to an asymmetric, unopposed pull of the orbicularis oris muscle. The cleft alar base is asymmetric and the cleft ala is displaced laterally, inferiorly, and posteriorly to its noncleft counterpart.[5] The nasal tip is also asymmetric, with the cleft side lower lateral cartilage (LLC) having a shorter medical crus and longer lateral crus than the LLC on the noncleft side (**Fig. 2**). The weakened and malpositioned cleft-side LLC produces a nostril that is wide and horizontally oriented.

The nasal septum in the unilateral cleft lip nose is deviated caudally to the noncleft side, and is bowed posteriorly to the cleft side (**Fig. 3**).[6] In a study of 140 nasal septa in patients with unilateral lip clefting, Crockett and Bumstead[7] found that the bony septum deviated into the cleft airway in 80% of these patients. Interestingly, most patients with clefting do not complain of nasal obstruction despite having significant deviation and

[a] Facial Plastic and Reconstructive Surgery, Department of Otolaryngology, University of California, Davis, 2521 Stockton Blvd., Suite 7200, Sacramento, CA 95817, USA
[b] Department of Otolaryngology, Asan Medical Center, University of Ulsan College of Medicine, 388-1 Pungnap-2dong, Songpa-gu, Seoul 138-736, Korea
* Corresponding author.
*E-mail address:* jonathan.sykes@ucdmc.ucdavis.edu (J.M. Sykes).

Facial Plast Surg Clin N Am 17 (2009) 133–144
doi:10.1016/j.fsc.2008.10.002

Box 1
Characteristics of unilateral cleft lip nasal deformity

Nasal tip

Medial crus of lower lateral cartilage shorter on cleft side

Lateral crus of lower lateral cartilage longer on cleft side (total length of lower lateral cartilage is same)

Lateral crus of lower lateral cartilage may be caudally displaced and may produce hooding of alar rim

Alar dome on cleft side is flat and displaced laterally

Columella

Short on cleft side

Base directed to noncleft side (secondary to contraction of orbicularis oris muscle)

Nostril

Horizontal orientation on cleft side

Alar base

Displaced laterally, posteriorly, and inferiorly

Nasal floor

Usually absent

Nasal septum

Caudal deflection to the noncleft side and posterior deviation to the cleft side

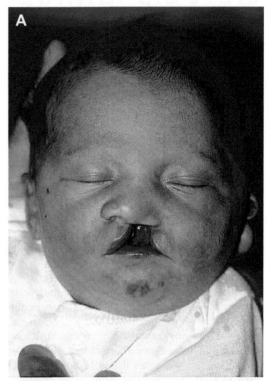

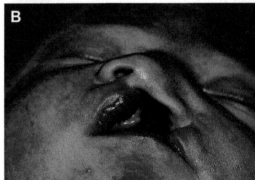

Fig. 1. Full face (A) and base (B) view of a 7-day-old child with a left unilateral cleft lip palate and deformity. The patient has obvious alar base asymmetry and deviation of the caudal nasal septum to the noncleft side.

abnormality of the nasal airway. In all likelihood, this tolerance of major abnormalities of the nasal septum can be attributed to the fact that cleft patients became use to their nasal airway anatomy and associated nasal breathing from a very young age.

The etiology of the asymmetry of the cleft alar base is a lack of skeletal support on the cleft-side alar base.[8] Deformities of the bony skeleton near the pyriform aperture result in inadequate support of the alar base both medially (at the columella) and laterally (at the alar-facial groove). The lack of medial and lateral support causes introversion of the nasal ala and webbing of the nasal vestibule (**Fig. 4**).[9] The contour of the lateral crus of the LLC is often concave, secondary to the lack of medial and lateral support. Introversion of the cleft ala is defined as a posterior and inferior malposition of the cephalic border of the lateral crus of the LLC. The combination of the lack of skeletal support and the malposition of the cleft

LLC causes weakness of the external nasal valve, often further compromising nasal breathing in the cleft patient.

The middle third of the nose in the unilateral cleft lip nasal deformity is also characterized by weakness of the upper lateral cartilages (ULC) and malposition of these cartilages.[6] Again, this weakness results from inadequate skeletal support and is often manifest by concave ULC. This weakness typically affects the internal nasal valve on the cleft side.

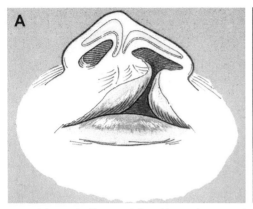
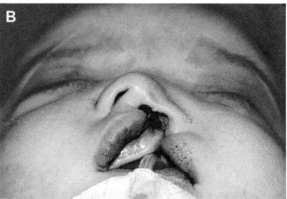

**Fig. 2.** Schematic diagram (*A*) and base photograph (*B*) of a left complete unilateral cleft and palate with obvious asymmetry of the alar base.

## Bilateral Cleft Nasal Deformity

The bilateral cleft lip nasal deformity is also caused by a lack of skeletal support. The bilateral cleft lip nose is usually not grossly asymmetric. Of course, if a marked difference exists on the two sides of the lip, there can be gross asymmetry of the cleft nasal tip and alar base in the bilateral cleft lip patient.

The bilateral cleft lip nose is characterized by a lack of skin and cartilaginous support in the nasal tip.[10] The columella in bilaterally deformities is typically short and there is inadequate projection of the nasal tip. The extent of columellar shortening is related to the size, shape, and position of the prolabium, and to the severity of the cleft deformity (**Fig. 5**). An abnormal junction between the columella and the central aspect of the upper lip

is usually present. Characteristics of the bilateral cleft lip nasal deformity are listed in **Box 2**.

The medial crura of the LLC are short, and the lateral crura are both long in bilateral clefts (**Fig. 6**). This results in underprojection of the nasal tip, and displacement of the alar bases in a posterior, lateral, and inferior location versus noncleft patients. If one side of the lip is more involved than the other side, the short columella is typically deviated toward the less involved side, pulling the tip toward that direction. The nostrils are more horizontal than those in noncleft patients. The nasal septum is usually midline, being deviated caudally to the less involved side if asymmetry exists. The middle nasal third exhibits poor cartilaginous support, compromising the internal nasal valve and affecting functional nasal breathing.

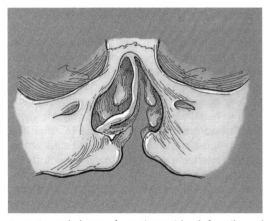

**Fig. 3.** Bony skeleton of a patient with a left unilateral cleft lip showing obvious deviation of the nasal septum to the noncleft side. The septum deviates to the noncleft side because of asymmetric pull of the unopposed orbicularis oris muscles.

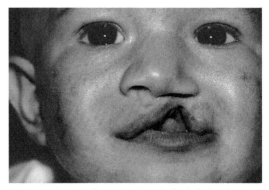

**Fig. 4.** Patient with incomplete left cleft lip showing obvious left nasal deformity with left alar hooding and webbing of the left nasal vestibule. The alar base is deviated posteriorly, inferiorly, and laterally when compared with the noncleft side.

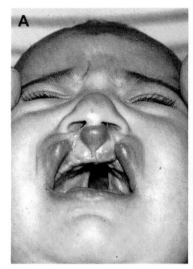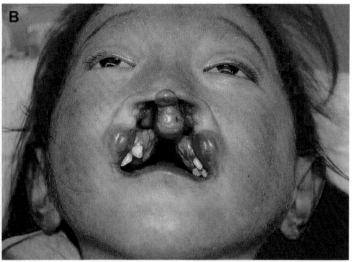

**Fig. 5.** Two base photographs of patients with bilateral cleft lip and palate deformities. (*A*) The lip clefting is incomplete and the columellar length is close to normal. (*B*) The manifestation of the cleft nasal deformity is much greater secondary to a very large complete cleft of the lip and palate with a "locked out" premaxilla and prolabium.

## TIMING AND PHILOSOPHY OF CLEFT NASAL RECONSTRUCTION

The decision to perform any nasal reconstructive surgery should take into account many factors, including the deformity itself, psychosocial effects on the child, and the impact of growth and surgical scarring. The advantages of early intervention in the cleft patient include minimizing the deformity during formative years, and lessening any asymmetries to allow symmetric nasal growth. The disadvantages of surgery before full nasal growth include creation of surgical scarring that may make any future nasal surgery more difficult. Additionally, early surgery may affect subsequent nasal growth.[1]

Cleft surgeons have shown some reluctance to operate on the nose before full nasal growth. This philosophy is a byproduct of experimental work that suggested that specific growth centers exist in the nose.[11,12] Interruption of these growth centers by either surgery or trauma was postulated to negatively affect nasal growth. However, there is no good clinical evidence to show that typical repositioning of cartilages and suture modification interferes with future nasal growth.[13]

Most cleft surgeons now think that early conservative intervention lessens the eventual secondary cleft nasal deformity.[14,15] Cleft tip rhinoplasty often minimizes nasal asymmetries and allows the nasal cartilages to grow in a symmetric fashion. For this reason, most surgeons perform primary cleft rhinoplasty to improve nasal tip and alar base symmetry. Also, primary nasal surgery on cleft

---

**Box 2**
**Characteristics of bilateral cleft lip nasal deformity**

Nasal tip

    Medial crura of LLC short bilaterally

    Lateral crura of LLC long bilaterally

    Lateral crura displaced caudally

    Alar domes poorly defined and widely separated, producing an amorphous tip

Columella

    Short

    Base is wide

Nostril

    Horizontal orientation bilaterally

Alar base

    Displaced laterally, posteriorly, and inferiorly

Nasal floor

    Usually absent bilaterally

Nasal septum

    In a complete bilateral cleft lip and palate, the septum is midline; however, if cleft on one side is incomplete, the septum deviates toward the less affected side

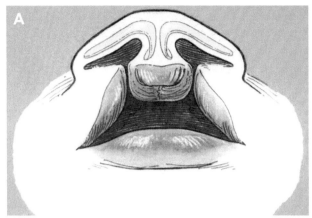
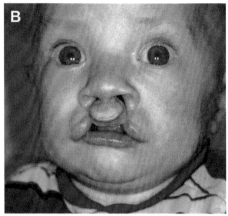

Fig. 6. Schematic diagram (A) and full face photograph (B) of a bilateral cleft lip deformity showing a short medial crus and a long lateral crus being longer then normal.

patients often obviates intermediate rhinoplasty. Additionally, the improved appearance associated with primary rhinoplasty creates psychological benefits for both the parents and the child.

## PRESURGICAL MANAGEMENT OF THE CLEFT NASAL DEFORMITY

The traditional approach to cleft management includes a single stage lip repair at 3 months of age, palatoplasty at approximately 1 year of age, alveolar bone grafting at 9 to 11 years, and definitive rhinoplasty at full facial growth. Nonsurgical repositioning of alveolar segments serves to lessen tension across the lip wound, improve nasal tip symmetry in wide unilateral clefts, and elongate the columella and expand the nasal soft tissues in bilateral clefts. Many reports have described presurgical devices designed to decrease the cleft gap and minimize the eventual lip and nasal deformity.[16,17] Presurgical nasoalveolar molding uses both an intraoral alveolar molding device and nasal molding prongs. Successful use of any presurgical orthopedic devices requires a team approach. This means a dedicated orthodontist, a flexible and patient surgeon, and an intelligent and compliant family. If properly performed, presurgical nasoalveolar molding can provide soft tissue expansion and mold the nasal infrastructure, thereby decreasing the nasal deformity (Fig. 7).

## PRIMARY CLEFT RHINOPLASTY

The goals of primary cleft nasal surgery are:[18]
Closure of the nasal floor and sill
Repositioning of the alar base
Repositioning of the lower lateral cartilages

In the unilateral deformity, cleft rhinoplasty is usually performed because noticeable asymmetry of the alar base and nasal tip is almost always

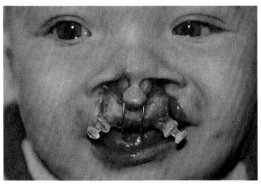

Fig. 7. Patient with a bilateral cleft lip deformity with presurgical and nasoalveolar molding device in position.

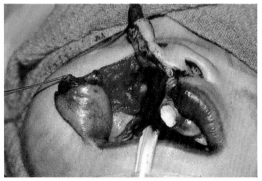

Fig. 8. Intraoperative photograph of a right complete cleft lip showing an external and internal alotomy freeing the alar base from its attachments to the inferior turbinate.

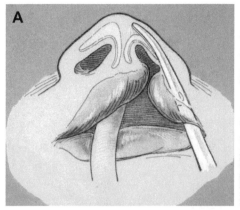
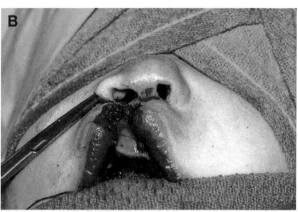

**Fig. 9.** Schematic diagram (*A*) and intraoperative photograph (*B*) of a patient with unilateral clefting showing unilateral dissection of the lower lateral cartilage from the external nasal skin.

present. In the bilateral deformity, asymmetry is usually not an issue, and primary rhinoplasty is often not performed. McComb and Coughlan[13] have shown in an 18-year individual study that nasal and midfacial growth were not significantly different in children who underwent primary cleft rhinoplasty versus age-matched normal and cleft controls who did not have primary rhinoplasty. Additionally, these investigators showed that the symmetry obtained with primary rhinoplasty was maintained into adult life.

### Technique

Primary cleft rhinoplasty can be accomplished by using the standard incisions typically used for lip repair.[18] No additional external incisions are typically necessary. The rotation advancement repair as described by Millard allows direct access to both the columella and the alar base. Some

investigators add intranasal incisions, such as the intercartilaginous or marginal incision, to reposition the LLC and to address alar hooding.

The first step in primary cleft rhinoplasty is to actively reposition the cleft alar base into an optimal three-dimensional position. This requires an internal alotomy to completely free the alar base attachment from the pyriform aperture (**Fig. 8**). An incision is made just lateral to the anterior attachment of the inferior turbinate. With adequate mobility, the alar base can be placed into a favorable, symmetric position.[8]

After mobilizing the cleft alar base or bases, the LLCs are freed from the external skin. A lateral tunnel is created with scissors dissection over the lateral crus to the nasal dome (**Fig. 9**). This tunnel is joined to a separate medial tunnel and the skin–soft tissue envelope is mobilized from the cartilaginous infrastructure (**Fig. 10**). If columellar lengthening is required on the cleft side, a back cut

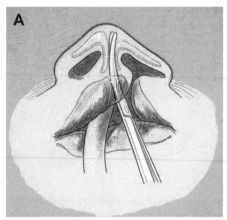
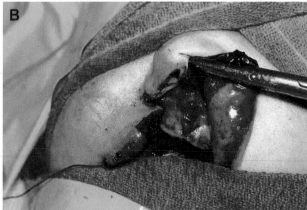

**Fig. 10.** Schematic diagram (*A*) and intraoperative photograph (*B*) showing medial dissection of the medial crus of the lower lateral cartilage from the columellar skin.

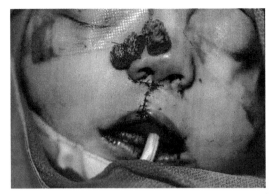

Fig. 11. Intraoperative photograph at the conclusion of the operation after nasal bolsters are applied to position the cleft alar cartilage in a more symmetric position verses the noncleft alar cartilage.

onto the columella with rotation of the c-flap into the opening may be performed.

After freeing the malpositioned alar base and dissecting the nasal tip cartilages, the floor of the nose is closed on the affected side. This provides medialization of the alar base in the unilateral cleft deformity. It is important not to make the cleft-side alar base too narrow. If the postsurgical cleft alar base is slightly wider than the non–cleft-side alar base, narrowing can easily be accomplished with a small excision of soft tissue at the nasal sill. However, if the cleft alar base is narrowed excessively, future widening is a difficult and imprecise procedure. Layered closure of the nasal floor also prevents nasolabial fistulae. The orbicularis oris muscle is carefully closed to provide further support to the floor of the nose.

After the lip is closed in meticulous layered fashion, the tip rhinoplasty is performed to reposition the LLC in a more symmetric position.[19] Repositioning the cartilages creates a new dome and

may be performed with either interdomal sutures or several nasal bolsters (**Fig. 11**). In the unilateral nasal deformity, a new dome is created in a more lateral position. The medial crus of the cleft LLC is lengthened and increased projection and tip support is obtained. The result is a more projected, defined, and symmetric nasal tip. If bolsters are used to perform the tip rhinoplasty, they are removed at 7 to 10 days postoperatively. If carefully performed, primary cleft rhinoplasty results in improved alar base symmetry and nasal tip definition (**Fig. 12**).

## SECONDARY CLEFT SEPTORHINOPLASTY

The secondary cleft nasal deformity is variable and is affected by the extent of the original abnormality and any prior surgeries performed.[20] Intermediate rhinoplasty is performed during childhood. The decision to perform nasal surgery before full nasal growth (intermediate rhinoplasty) is often made when the deformity is great enough to be associated with ridicule during adolescence.

Definitive septorhinoplasty is performed after full nasal growth and is typically done at age 15 in females and 17 in males. In cleft patients with significant dentofacial deformities (typically class III malocclusion and malar hypoplasia), definitive rhinoplasty is usually delayed until after the orthognathic surgery is completed. The goals of septorhinoplasty are to maximize functional nasal breathing and to optimize nasal and facial appearance. In most cases, the skeletal foundation, both dental and craniofacial, should be stabilized before performing definitive nasal surgery.

## DEFINITIVE CLEFT SEPTORHINOPLASTY

Although an endonasal approach may be used for cleft septorhinoplasty, the external, or open, approach is preferred. The external approach

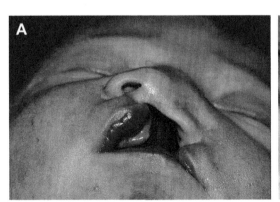

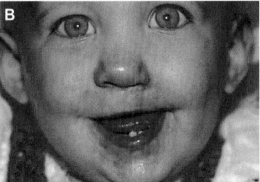

Fig. 12. (*A*) Two-day-old patient with obvious left cleft alar deformity and cleft nasal base asymmetry. (*B*) The same patient at 10 months of age after a unilateral rotation advancement cleft lip repair and primary tip rhinoplasty.

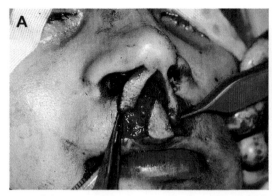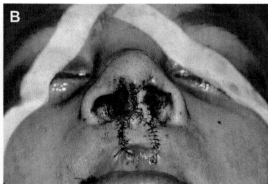

Fig. 13. (*A*) Intraoprative photograph of a patient with bilateral cleft lip showing forked flaps used to advance and augment the columellar skin and lengthen nasal tip projection. (*B*) The same patient after suturing the forked flaps into position and demonstrating lengthening of the columellar.

allows maximal visualization for diagnosis, and adequate exposure for placement and suturing of structural grafts.

If the amount of skin is deficient in the columella, skin and soft tissue can be advanced from the lip into the nose. In the unilateral cleft nasal deformity with a short columella, a V-to-Y lip skin advancement can be used to increase columellar soft tissue. In the bilateral cleft nasal deformity, additional columellar lengthening can be obtained with either a central V-to-Y skin advancement, or with upper lip forked flaps[21] (**Fig. 13**). If columellar soft tissue is sufficient, a standard inverted notched "V" incision is used to facilitate the external approach.

For the nasal septum, an endonasal approach using a hemitransfixion incision may be performed. Alternately, the nasal septum may be treated through an external approach by separating the soft tissue attachments of the medial crura

of the LLC, or superiorly by dividing the ULC attachments to the nasal septum.[6]

## NASAL SEPTOPLASTY

Correcting septal deformities in the cleft patient is an important initial maneuver. Septoplasty serves to relieve functional nasal obstruction and provide cartilage for graft material during the rhinoplasty. Additionally, nasal septal reconstruction allows three-dimensional nasal base symmetry and support to be established.

To reconstruct the caudal septum, the septomaxillary ligaments must be divided and a strip of inferior cartilage usually must be removed. The caudal septum is then moved into the midline and sutured into position with an anchoring suture to the nasal spine.[6] If there is an intrinsic convexity or concavity to the nasal septum, structural

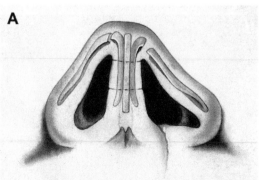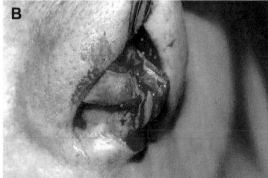

Fig. 14. (*A*) Schematic diagram of a left unilateral cleft lip with a columellar strut and dome suture to maximize nasal tip and columellar symmetry. (*B*) Intraoperative photograph of a patient with a columellar strut sutured into position to create three-dimensional symmetry.

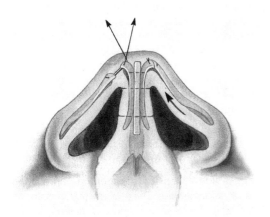

Fig. 15. Reconstitution of the cleft alar cartilage demonstrating stealing from the lateral crus to enhance nasal tip projection on the cleft side.

grafting is performed to straighten the deformity and provide caudal support.

## DEFINITIVE RHINOPLASTY

After stabilizing the caudal nasal septum and providing three-dimensional alar base symmetry, attention is turned to the external nasal form. Usually, symmetry and support of the nasal tip is established by placing a columellar cartilaginous strut graft.[22] The strut is placed between the medial crura and is designed to support and stabilize the tip and to create increased nasal tip projection (Fig. 14). It is important to establish three-dimensional nasal tip symmetry. In the unilateral deformity, the medial crus of the LLC is advanced in

the anterior-posterior dimension to equalize tip symmetry between the cleft and noncleft sides. Additionally, the cleft-side alar cartilage is elevated superiorly versus the non–cleft-side LLC to alleviate alar hooding.

Once the nasal tip is stabilized with the columellar strut, other tip maneuvers are performed to improve nasal tip definition and symmetry. An LLC steal is performed to increase projection on the cleft-side alar cartilage. The LLC steal can be performed with only suturing, or can involve vertically dividing the LLC lateral to the existing surgical dome. The intent of the LLC steal is to recruit cartilage from the lateral crus of the LLC, and give it to the medial crus of that side. This maneuver lengthens the medial crus, adding projection to the affected side. Reconstitution of the divided LLC is always performed to reestablish cartilaginous alar support (Fig. 15). By vertically dividing (and reconstituting) the LLC at different points, nasal tip symmetry can be achieved and projection can be enhanced.[23]

If there is a residual alar hooding of the cleft-side cartilage after completing the LLC division and reconstitution, the LLC can be sutured to the ULC to reposition the alar rim more superiorly (Fig. 16). After these tip techniques are completed, a cartilaginous tip graft may be placed. Tip grafts are added to improve tip support and definition, and to camouflage residual tip asymmetries and irregularities. The cartilaginous grafts are fashioned from nasal septal cartilage and sutured to the existing medial crural framework.

The middle one-third of the nose in cleft patients often is weak, creating both aesthetic and functional (internal nasal valve) deformities. These

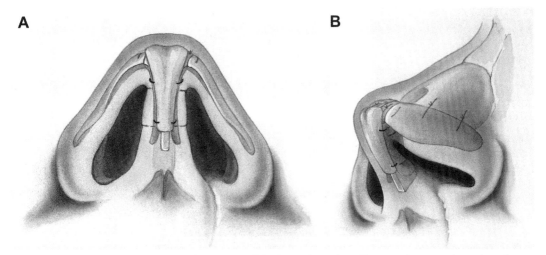

Fig. 16. (A and B) Suturing of the cephalic margin of the lower lateral cartilage to the upper lateral cartilage to diminish alar hooding on the cleft side.

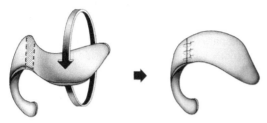

**Fig. 17.** Flipping of a concave alar cartilage to create a convex shape to the cartilage.

middle-third cartilaginous deficiencies may be treated with onlay grafts, spreader grafts to the internal nasal valve, or flaring sutures.[24] In the unilateral cleft deformity, subtle asymmetry of the middle nasal third often exists, requiring the use of a unilateral spreader graft placed between the nasal septum and upper lateral cartilage.

The bony vault of the cleft nose is treated in a standard fashion. Hump reduction and medial osteotomies, with or without lateral osteotomies are performed as needed. These are accomplished to straighten and narrow the nasal bridge and align the nasal profile.

## TREATMENT OF THE MALPOSITIONED ALAR RIM

The cleft-side alar cartilage is poorly supported and always malpositioned. The etiology of this malposition is lack of alar base support. Deficiency in alar base support causes lack of projection of the cleft-side alar cartilage. In addition, the LLC has an altered contour secondary to the lack of support.

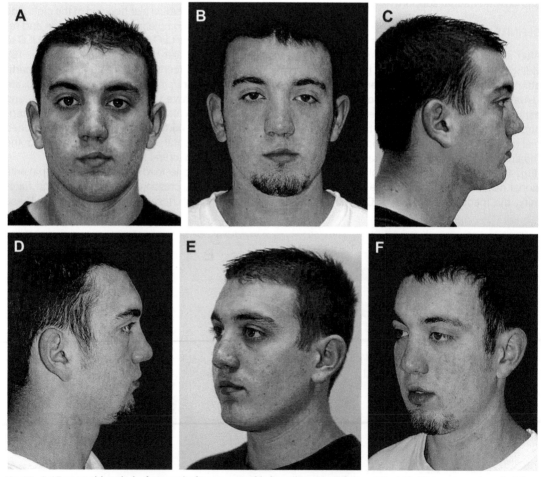

**Fig. 18.** A 17-year-old male before and after repair of left unilateral cleft lip with definitive external septorhinoplasty. (*A*) Preoperative frontal view. (*B*) Postoperative frontal view. (*C*) Preoperative right lateral view. (*D*) Postoperative right lateral view. (*E*) Preoperative left oblique view. (*F*) Postoperative left oblique view.

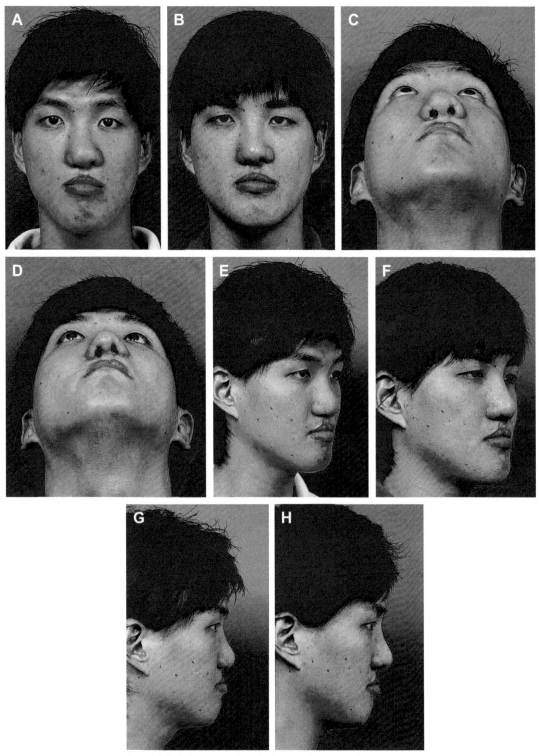

Fig. 19. A patient with a bilateral cleft lip and palate before and after definitive open septorhinoplasty. (*A*) Preoperative frontal view. (*B*) Postoperative frontal view. (*C*) Preoperative basal view. (*D*) Postoperative basal view. (*E*) Preoperative right oblique view. (*F*) Postoperative right oblique view. (*G*) Preoperative right lateral view. (*H*) Postoperative right lateral view.

The cleft-side lateral crus of the LLC is concave, contributing to the introverted alar contour.[25,26]

Treatment of the concave lateral crus of the LLC can be accomplished with various methods. The cartilage can be dissected from the underlying vestibular skin, flipped, and replaced with the convex side outward (**Fig. 17**). Another technique involves placing an alar strut graft between the existing concave LLC and the vestibular skin. This underlay cartilage graft strengthens the lateral crus of the LLC and changes the concave nature of the cartilage.

Lastly, horizontal mattress sutures can be placed to change the concave lateral crus into a convex orientation. Whatever the technique used, the goal of these maneuvers is to change the concave alar cartilage into a convex one, improving the contour of the alar rim and the function of the external nasal valve.[25]

## SUMMARY

Reconstruction of cleft lip nose is extremely challenging. The congenital malformation involves all tissue layers, from skeletal platform to external nasal skin. Primary rhinoplasty is used to maximize nasal symmetry and minimize psychological ridicule for the child. This also allows the nose to grow in a symmetric fashion. Definitive rhinoplasty is performed using an external rhinoplasty approach. Structural grafting is employed to maximize function, structure, support, and symmetry (**Figs. 18 and 19**).

## REFERENCES

1. Sykes JM, Senders CW. Surgery of the cleft lip and nasal deformity. Oper Tech Otolaryngol Head Neck Surg 1990;1:219–24.
2. Sykes JM. Senders CW. Pathologic anatomy of cleft lip, palate and nasal deformity. In: Meyers AD, editor. Biological basis of facial plastic surgery. New York: Thieme 1993, p. 57–71.
3. Blair VP. Nasal deformities associated with congenital cleft of the lip. JAMA 1925;84:185–7.
4. Huffman WC, Lierle DM. Studies on the pathologic anatomy of the unilateral hare-lip nose. Plast Reconstr Surg 1949;4:225–34.
5. Avery JK. The nasal capsule in cleft palate. Anat Anz 1962;109(Suppl):722.
6. Jablon JH, Sykes JM. Nasal airway problems in the cleft lip population. Facial Plast Surg Clin North AM 1999;7:391–403.
7. Crockett D, Bumstead R. Nasal airway, otologic and audiologic problems associated with cleft lip and palate. In: Bardack J, Morris HL, editors. Multidisciplinary management of cleft lip and palate. Philadelphia: WB Saunders; 1990.
8. Sykes JM, Senders CW. Surgical treatment of the unilateral cleft nasal deformity at the time of lip repair. Facial Plast Surg Clin North Am 1995;3:69–77.
9. Stenstrom SJ. The alar cartilage and the nasal deformity in unilateral cleft lip. Plast Reconstr Surg 1966; 38:223–31.
10. Cronin TD. The bilateral cleft lip with bilateral cleft of the primary palate. In: Converse JM, editor. Reconstructive plastic surgery. Philadelphia: WB Saunders; 1964.
11. Sarnat BG, Wexler MR. Growth of the face and jaws after resection of the septal cartilage in the rabbit. Am J Anat 1996;118:755–67.
12. Bernstein L. Early submucous resection of nasal septal cartilage: a pilot study in canine pups. Arch Otolaryngol 1973;97:272–85.
13. McComb HK, Coghlan BA. Primary repair of the unilateral cleft lip nose: completion of a longitudinal study. Cleft Palate Craniofac J 1996;33:23–31.
14. Mulliken JB, Martinez-Perez D. The principle of rotation advancement for the repair of unilateral complete cleft lip and nasal deformity: technical variations and analysis of results. Plast Reconstr Surg 1999;104:1247–9.
15. TerKonda RP, Sykes JM. Controversies and advances in unilateral cleft lip repair. Curr Opin Otolaryngol Head Neck Surg 1997;5:223–7.
16. Grayson BH, Santiago PE, Beecht LE, Cutting CB. Presurgical nasoalveolar molding in infants with cleft lip and palate. Cleft Palate Craniofac J 1999;36: 486–98.
17. Liou EJW, Subramanian M, Chen PKT, et al. The progressive changes of nasal symmetry and growth after nasoalveolar molding: a three-year follow-up study. Plast Reconstr Surg 2004;114:858–64.
18. Ness JA, Sykes JM. Basics of Millard rotation-advancement technique for repair of the unilateral cleft lip deformity. Facial Plast Surg 1993;9:167–76.
19. Salyer KE, Genecov ER, Genecov DG. Unilateral cleft lip-nose repair: a thirty three-year experience. J Craniofac Surg 2003;14:549–58.
20. Gilles HD, Kilner TP. Hare-lip: operation for correction of secondary deformities. Lancet 1932;223:1369–75.
21. Millard Dr Jr. Columella lengthening by a forked flap. Plast Reconstr Surg 1958;22:545.
22. Sykes JM, Senders CW, Wang TD, et al. Use of the open approach for repair of secondary cleft lip-nasal deformities. Facial Plast Surg 1993;1:111–26.
23. Toruumi DM, Johnson CM. Open structure rhinoplasty. Facial Plast Surg Clin North Am 1993;1:1–22.
24. Park SS. Treatment of the internal nasal valve. Facial Plast Surg 1999;7:333–45.
25. Park BY, Lew DH, Lee YH. A comparative study of the lateral crus of alar cartilage in unilateral cleft lip nasal deformity. Plast Reconstr Surg 1998;101:905–19.
26. Chand MS, Toriumi DM. Treatment of the external nasal valve. Facial Plast Surg 1999;7:347–55.

# Complications in Rhinoplasty

J. Jared Christophel, MD, Stephen S. Park, MD, FACS*

**KEYWORDS**

• Rhinoplasty • Complications • Etiology • Prevention

Rhinoplasty can be a rewarding surgery for the patient and doctor, impacting patient self-esteem and quality of life. When outcomes are positive, it is easy to consider the procedure straight-forward and predictable. After complications arise, especially years later, the deformities can be extremely challenging to correct and they may create angst for even the experienced surgeon. The complex interplay of soft tissue and structural framework makes surgical manipulations difficult and sometimes unpredictable. In addition to the technical rigor, patients seeking aesthetic rhinoplasties are often keenly aware of their appearance and scrutinize even subtle imperfections. This combination of factors makes rhinoplasty a high stakes surgery.

Although immediate postoperative complications, such as bleeding and infection, are always a risk, this article discusses primarily the more complex and problematic outcomes. Ascertaining complications in cosmetic rhinoplasty is difficult given the subjective nature of the aesthetic result. One might expect patients who seek rhinoplasty to be more critical of the results, but our experience and that of others show that the surgeon is more apt to be dissatisfied than the patient.[1]

One method of defining complications is to look at the rate of revision or secondary rhinoplasty. The literature quotes an average rate of revision surgery of 8%–15%, with some expert series requiring revision in 5%–10% of primary cases.[2,3] Complications can be classified by their anatomic etiology, such as buckled cartilage or soft tissue collapse.[4] Although useful in describing the defect, this anatomic grouping fails to delineate which principle of primary rhinoplasty was violated.

Another useful way to view complications in rhinoplasty is to consider the technical pitfalls in primary surgery that can lead to untoward long-term results. Although not a treatise on how to correct each complication, this discussion will center on what complications occur after primary rhinoplasty and how they could have been avoided with proper planning and execution. **Table 1** summarizes the high points of this discussion for easy reference.

## DORSAL HUMP REDUCTION

Reducing a large dorsal hump may be the most common specific aim for primary rhinoplasty. This task is often viewed by patients, and occasionally surgeons, as simple and straight-forward, yet aesthetic and functional complications can easily arise. The nasal dorsum consists of a bony upper vault and a cartilaginous middle vault. Patients with a prominent dorsal hump generally have an excess of both, and attempts to reduce the hump often involve osteotomies, rasping, and/or grafting. When attempting to reduce a dorsal hump, one must be aware of the pitfalls that lead to each of the following deformities.

### Pollybeak Deformity

A pollybeak is cited as being one of the most common deformities encountered after primary rhinoplasty, with most series quoting 40%–64% of the cases for which secondary rhinoplasty was performed.[5–7] The appearance of a pollybeak is created when the supratip projects beyond the tip in the plane of the nasal dorsum. This gives the nose a bulbous, rounded shape with the illusion of tip ptosis due to the absence of a supratip break (**Fig. 1**).

Division of Facial Plastic and Reconstructive Surgery, Department of Otololaryngology–Head and Neck Surgery, University of Virginia Health System, PO Box 800713, Charlottesville, VA 22908-0713, USA
* Corresponding author.
*E-mail address:* SSP8a@virginia.edu (S.S. Park).

Facial Plast Surg Clin N Am 17 (2009) 145–156
doi:10.1016/j.fsc.2008.09.012
1064-7406/08/$ – see front matter © 2009 Elsevier Inc. All rights reserved.

facialplastic.theclinics.com

**Table 1**
Summary of complications associated with the primary rhinoplasty goal and the surgical principles that will prevent their formation

| Rhinoplasty Goal | Complication | Etiology | How to Prevent |
|---|---|---|---|
| **Dorsal hump reduction** | Pollybeak | Failure to resect anterior septal angle | Ensure adequate resection of dorsal septum |
| | Excessive resection | Scooping of cartilage or plunging osteotomies | Conservative resection and leave biplanar dorsum with slight hump under thin skin of rhinion. |
| | Open roof | Medial aspect of nasal bones remaining flared and lateral | Lateral osteotomies |
| | Inverted-V | See above. See below. | See above. See below. |
| | Internal valve collapse | Disarticulation of ULC from dorsal septum | Middle vault reconstruction with fixation of ULC back to septum; consider spreader grafts |
| **Dorsal augmentation** | Alloplast extrusion | Foreign body reaction | Avoidance |
| | Allogenic resorption | Lack of viability and autoimmune | Avoidance |
| | Autogenous warping | Natural tendency over time | Carving central core of rib cartilage and rigid fixation |
| **Twisted Dorsum** | Persistent Deformity | Intrinsic Nasal Bone Deformity | Intermediate osteotomies |
| | | Frontal Beak Deviation | 2 mm percutaneous horizontal osteo. |
| | | Middle Vault Twisting | Splinting; resection and reimplantation of dorsal septum |
| **Tip Narrowing** | Alar Retraction | Wound contracture | Minimize resection |
| | Inter-Valve area Collapse | Contracture and collapse from binding sutures | Minimize resection; Strut grafting to straighten intrinsic recurvature of LLC |
| | Bossae | Contracture and buckling of LLC | Minimize resection; camouflage graft |
| | Pinched Tip | Over-aggressive narrowing from sutures and resection | Maintain adequate space between tip defining points |
| | Excessive Cephalic Rotation | Over-resection of LLC | Minimize resection; careful with dome binding sutures |
| | Tip Ptosis | Loss of tip support | Recreation of tip ligaments with suture |
| | Inadequate Definition | Thick skin, lack of projection, and reliance on resection | Over projection through thicker skin envelope |

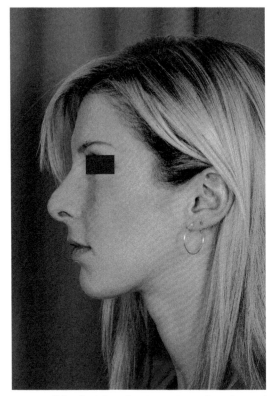

Fig. 1. Pollybeak deformity. Supratip projects beyond the tip in the plane of the nasal dorsum.

Multiple etiologies can lead to a pollybeak deformity, but two of the most common causes are: the inadequate resection of the supratip dorsum, specifically the anterior septal angle; and the disruption of tip support leading to postoperative tip depression.[6,8,9] To prevent the formation of a pollybeak, the surgeon must ensure adequate resection of the dorsal septum at the end of the operation by palpating the dorsum with the soft tissue envelope re-draped. The major tip support mechanisms of the nose, including the inherent integrity of the lower lateral cartilages (LLC) and the fibrous attachment of the medial crura to the caudal septum, must be re-established during rhinoplasty as scarring and contracture will lead to formation of a pollybeak with time.[10]

Another less common cause is the accumulation of scar tissue in the supratip region following dorsal reduction. This scenario can be improved with conservative steroid injections to the dorsum.[11]

## Excessive Resection

When attempting to reduce a dorsal hump that involves both the cartilaginous and bony nasal dorsum, inadvertent over-resection can leave a "scooped out" appearance of the middle third from a lateral view. (Fig. 2) Excessive resection

of the septum can leave a similar appearance over time due to the classic saddle nose deformity, but must be distinguished from over-resection of the dorsum as the primary fault.[12] In addition to the loss of dorsal height, excessive resection can cause simultaneous inverted-V and open roof deformities from an anterior view. These are discussed separately.

This problem is more common in patients with short nasal bones in whom simultaneous osteotomies are performed: if the bones form the hypotenuse of a right angle triangle, they must medialize further after dorsal resection and thus lose more height (dorsal projection). Excessive resection can also be avoided by keeping in mind the variable thickness of the skin of the nasal dorsum. When reducing a hump, the plane of resection must be slightly biphasic, taking care to leave a slight hump at the rhinion where the skin is thinnest.

### Open Roof Deformity

Over-resection of the bony nasal dorsum can lead to an open roof deformity. The nasal bridge appears widened and artificially flat. A cross-section of the upper third would reveal a trapezoidal

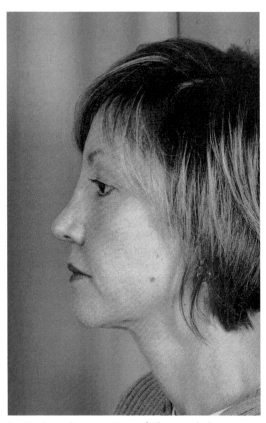

Fig. 2. Excessive resection of the nasal dorsum can leave a "scooped out" appearance.

appearance instead of a gently curved triangle. At times, the dorsal septum can be palpated, or even observed, projecting between the nasal bones.

This is due to inadequate medialization of the nasal bones, usually due to improper osteotomy technique. The lateral osteotomies may be incomplete at their cephalic end; there may be only a greenstick fracture which prevents complete mobilization; or the dorsal reduction may have left a wedge of nasal bone between the septum and lateral wall at the cephalic portion.[6] Patients with a narrow nasal base, but broad dorsum, may only require a medial oblique osteotomy to reduce an open roof.[13]

To ensure adequate medialization of the nasal bones after dorsal hump reduction, the surgeon must feel the nasal bones in-fracture after the lateral osteotomy and re-drape the soft tissue envelope and palpate with a moistened gloved finger to appreciate any residual "open" component to the dorsum.

### Inverted-V

The inverted-V deformity, also known as an inverted pyramid deformity, describes the sharp transition between the cephalic border of a narrowed middle vault with the caudal end of the nasal bones. There are multiple causes of this inverted-V deformity, but the final anatomic etiology is the same: the upper lateral cartilages (ULCs) are often displaced medially with respect to the nasal bones.[14] The caudal border of the bones and the shadow they create give rise to a visible inverted-V and a disruption of the brow–tip aesthetic line. (**Fig. 3**) Patients with short nasal bones and long upper lateral cartilages seem disposed to this inverted-V problem.[4]

There are two primary reasons for the development of this anatomic deformity. The first reason is a failure to medialize the nasal bones after dorsal reduction, leaving them lateral and visible. Second is the relationship of the ULCs to the dorsal septum. The ULCs may become destabilized from one another with subsequent medial collapse over time. In addition, the new dorsal septum that is created by virtue of the hump resection is narrower than the original, native dorsum. (**Fig. 4**A, B) Even if the ULCs scar firmly to the septum, they will create a pinched middle vault area.

Prevention of this common deformity is accomplished by completion lateral osteotomies following resection of the upper third and adequate closure of the open roof. Middle vault reconstruction is imperative following a reduction of the dorsal septum. This is facilitated by preservation of the mucoperichondrium at the junction of the

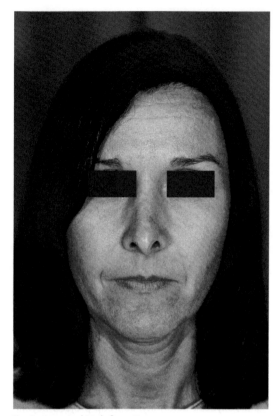

Fig. 3. Inverted-V deformity.

ULC and dorsal septum.[1] Further reinforcement comes from direct suture suspension of the ULCs back to the dorsal septum. Following an aggressive resection in this area, the new dorsal septum will require prophylactic spreader grafts to recreate the natural flare seen in the native dorsal septum (**Fig. 5**).

### Internal Valve Collapse/Hourglass Deformity

The internal nasal valve refers to the intranasal area between the ULC and the dorsal septum.[14] As mentioned above in the inverted-V discussion, any maneuver that weakens the support of the ULC and dorsal septum, such as resecting a dorsal hump, can lead to progressive displacement and a pinched middle vault. This is the same anatomic problem that leads to the formation of an inverted-V as mentioned above; however, in patients with a normal width of the bony dorsum, the pinched middle vault will show a less marked transition, often referred to as an hourglass deformity. In addition to creating the cosmetic deformity of an hourglass due to disruption of the brow tip aesthetic line, collapse of the ULC can cause functional airway obstruction at the area of the internal nasal valve.

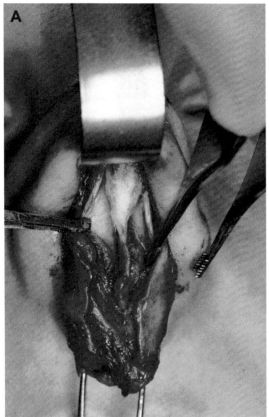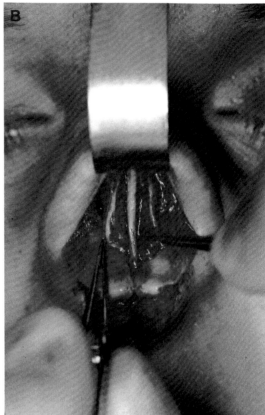

**Fig. 4.** The native dorsum (*A*) has a natural dorsal flair that is lost once resected, leaving the new narrower nasal dorsum (*B*).

Again, preservation of the ventral mucoperichondrial envelope when performing the dorsal reduction will help to prevent this. Some surgeons prefer to separate the ULC from the dorsal septum before performing the dorsal reduction to ensure the preservation of the mucoperichondrial envelope at the internal nasal valve.[15,16] This method requires resuspending the ULC to the dorsal septum by using either spreader grafts, butterfly grafts, or flaring sutures.[17]

## DORSAL AUGMENTATION

The surgeon planning to perform dorsal augmentation can choose from alloplastic, allogenic, or autogenous grafts. Surgeon preference can be based on the anatomic region being augmented, donor availability, or anecdotal experience, but each class is associated with a host of potential complications.

### Alloplastic Grafts

There are multiple alloplastic implants available for use in facial plastic surgery. The most commonly used substances include Gore-Tex (WL Gore,

Newark, DE), Silastic (Dow Corning Corp, Midland, MI), and Medpor (Porex Medical, Newnan, GA).

Expanded polytetrafluoroethylene (Gore-Tex) has been used as an implant in facial plastic surgery for the last 25 years.[18] Its unique pore size allows tissue ingrowth, but theoretically prevents bacterial colonization. The substance is pliable, and therefore is better suited to smooth soft tissue irregularities rather than to provide structure.[19] Further, it does not resorb. The literature quotes infection rates from 2.5% to 3.2% in large series.[20,21] There is a clear difference in infection rate when it is used in primary rhinoplasty (1.2%–1.4%) versus revision rhinoplasty (4.6%–5.4%). Most infections occur in a delayed fashion (>6 months), and almost all grafts that become infected will require removal (**Figs. 6** and **7**).[21]

Silastic is an organic polymer composed of silicone–oxygen chains that are cross-linked by methyl side groups. The amount of cross-linking determines the rigidity of the implant. Like Gore-Tex, it does not resorb over time. Unlike Gore-Tex, it is a solid, nonporous material, and does not permit tissue ingrowth. Therefore, it is prone to mobility and a higher extrusion rate. The rate

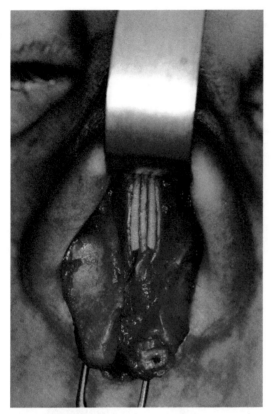

Fig. 5. Dorsal spreader grafts in place to recreate dorsal width.

of extrusion can be as high as 50% if it is used in the columella and 10% if used on the nasal dorsum.[22]

Medpor is a more rigid implant composed of high density porous polyethylene. Its pores average 200 microns and are arranged in a lattice configuration. This allows bone and soft tissue to integrate, providing stabilization to the surrounding tissue. It has a similar extrusion rate to that of Gore-Tex.[23]

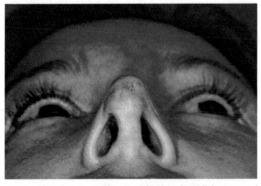

Fig. 6. Alloplastic implant with skin breakdown and rejection.

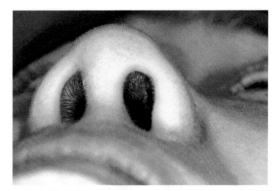

Fig. 7. Alloplastic implant extruding intranasally with recurrent infections.

Should an alloplastic implant extrude or become infected and require removal, immediate reconstruction with allogenic or autogenous rib has been successful.[24,25]

### Allogenic Grafts

Allogenic grafts, sometimes called homografts, are tissue taken from another animal of the same species. Commonly used allogenic grafts in rhinoplasty include irradiated homograft costal cartilage (IHCC) and AlloDerm (LifeCell Corp., Woodlands, TX).

Irradiated rib tends to have lower rates of infection requiring removal compared with alloplasts, but it has a higher rate of resorption, with 3%–11% of grafts having cosmetically significant resorption.[26,27]

AlloDerm is an acellular dermal graft derived from cadaveric skin. Because it is acellular, it does not illicit an immune response, which is thought to be the reason for its low infection rate. It is often used for contour abnormalities in patients with thin skin.[28]

### Autogenous Grafts

Autogenous material represents the ideal graft choice in terms of immunogenicity and infection rate. Although they have the obvious downside of donor site morbidity, the larger grafts are also plagued by warping. The most common sources for use in rhinoplasty include septal cartilage, auricular cartilage, costal cartilage, and calvarial bone. Auricular and septal cartilage have a very low resorption rate and time is thought to increase their purpose by fibrosis and scarring.[29] Costal cartilage is often preferred for use in large nasal reconstructions requiring significant dorsal or collumelar support. (**Fig. 8**A) It has a much lower rate of resorption than irradiated homograft rib, but it does suffer from a tendency to warp with time.

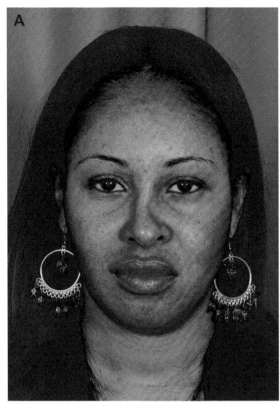
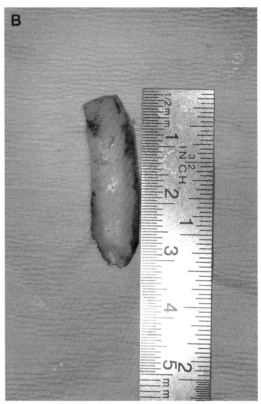

Fig. 8. (A) A posttraumatic deformity of the nasal dorsum in need of structural grafting. (B) an intraoperative photo of the patient's concentrically carved rib, set aside for 90 minutes in saline to assess warping.

This can be avoided if the graft is carved in a concentric manner from the donor rib.[30] The graft can also be set aside in sterile saline during surgery to interrogate its warping potential (**Fig. 8B**).

## TWISTED DORSUM

Managing the twisted nose is one of the most difficult problems in aesthetic rhinoplasty. The most common complication from this type of rhinoplasty is a persistent postoperative deviation. This is usually due either an intrinsic deformity of the nasal bones, frontal beak deviation, or middle vault twisting. Whether a persistent deformity is considered a complication of the surgery, or failure to correctly recognize the underlying anatomic deformity, remains debatable. There are circumstances where severe twisting and deviations will recur, perhaps due to the memory of the framework or soft tissue, and a repeat "touch-up" can be expected.

### Intrinsic Deformity of Nasal Bones

Should an underlying intrinsic deformity of the nasal bones go unrecognized before rhinoplasty, traditional osteotomies will uniformly fail because the mobilized bones are themselves twisted. It is critical to palpate the bones carefully and determine if they are symmetric and straight. If intrinsic deviations are detected, such as occurs from prior nasal fractures, they will usually require multiple osteotomies, including intermediate osteotomies between the medial and lateral ones.

### Frontal Beak Deviation

The frontal beak can also be deviated to the side from previous trauma. The typical flaring medial osteotomies will not mobilize that triangular segment and they can hinder a complete bony realignment. This segment will require complete mobilization through a direct fracture across the nasion, usually performed with a 2-mm percutaneous osteotome. The "rocker deformity" is created by osteotomies that extend too far superiorly. This can be avoided by performing osteotomies along a natural cleavage plane where the nasal bone gradually thickens in the cephalic and medial directions.[31] Secondary correction requires completion percutaneous osteotomies to create smaller bony segments and more complete reduction.

## Middle Vault Twisting

Middle vault reduction can also create a twisted deformity following hump resection. This occurs as the hump is reduced and a new dorsal septum is created. This area was previously intranasal and represented the intranasal dorsal septum. After an aggressive hump reduction is performed, it may unmask an occult twisted septum and create an iatrogenic twisted nose. This is best anticipated preoperatively via careful intranasal inspection and anticipation of the possible need to straighten the septum with splints or camouflage grafts. If the twisting of the septum is severe, it may require resection and re-implantation. Asymmetry to the ULC's is uncommon but can also give rise to subtle deviations across the dorsum.

## TIP NARROWING

There are many published methods of surgically altering the nasal tip. These have likely evolved because of the complex relationship of the soft tissue and underlying structure in the tip region. Accordingly, there are more potential complications in the tip than anywhere else in the nose. Many of these complications can be avoided with proper surgical planning.

## Alar Retraction

The usual culprit behind alar retraction is scarring of the LLC superiorly, thus creating a contour abnormality across the alar rim (**Fig. 9**).

The most common etiology of this is overly aggressive resection of the existing LLCs in an attempt to refine the tip lobule. The dead space that is created is subject to continued, long-term contracture and the ultimate retraction of the lateral crus and alar rim notching. Rhinoplasty incisions used to gain access to the nose, particularly the rim incision or a poorly placed marginal incision, are other potential causes.[14,32]

Preservation of a strong support to the alar rim is paramount for prevention of this characteristic stigma. Rather than resect tip structure and support, the contemporary philosophy is more akin to reshaping with sutures.

## Intervalve Area Collapse

Much of the published literature on post-rhinoplasty nasal obstruction focuses on the internal nasal valve and the contribution of the ULCs as mentioned above. The intervalve area refers to an area between the external and internal valves, immediately lateral to the lateral crura, corresponding to the supra-alar crease. This critical area is naturally devoid of cartilaginous support

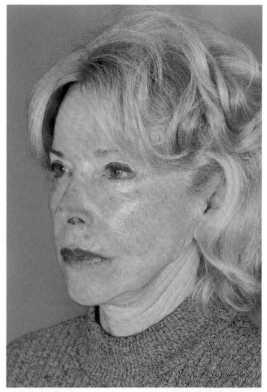

**Fig. 9.** Alar rim retraction due to previous over-resection of lateral crus.

and subject to collapse from tip maneuvers, including the cartilage-sparing dome-binding sutures. It is in precisely this area that most functional batten grafts are placed.[17] If attempting to increase tip rotation or reduce bulbosity with a cephalic trim, care must be taken to leave 7 to 9 millimeters of lateral crus, or over-resection will lead to intervalve collapse.

Common tip-narrowing procedures such as dome-binding sutures can create iatrogenic nasal obstruction due to subtle malformations of the lateral crura. Occult recurvature or a paradoxical concavity to the lateral crus can predispose to obstruction at the intervalve area following tip sutures. (**Fig. 10**) The amount of LLC recurvature must be assessed preoperatively, and if the planned tip maneuver will medialize the lateral crus or exacerbate the recurvature, then consideration should be given to placing lateral crural strut grafts.[33] Similarly, the concave crus should be noted during the initial evaluation.

A vertically-oriented lower lateral crus, often referred to as a parenthesis deformity, can also predispose a patient to collapse at the intervalve area. These patients have an inherent weakness in the lateral wall, and any resection of the lateral crura will diminish what little cartilaginous support exists.

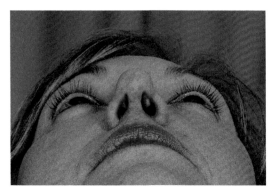

**Fig. 10.** A patient being evaluated for secondary rhinoplasty for nasal obstruction, here shown with recurvature of the LLC.

## Bossae

Bossae are protruding contour deformities of the nasal tip due to irregularities in the lower lateral cartilages. In one large series, lower third abnormalities were the most common reason for revision surgery, of which bossae were second only to pollybeak.[34] It is one of the more common complications of primary rhinoplasty and can occur in up to 4% of patients postoperatively.[35] Some surgeons divide bossae into two categories: early and late. Early bossae are seen soon after surgery and are due to abnormalities of the LLC. Late bossae usually appear a few years after surgery and are due to fibrosis and scarring over a weakened cartilaginous framework.[36]

Certain patients carry a higher risk for forming bossae postoperatively. Females, young patients, patients with thin skin, and those with a bifid nasal tip have a tendency to develop bossae when undergoing the same maneuvers as other patients.[35]

Early bossae are more likely to form if there is asymmetric alignment of the domes of the LLC at the end of the initial rhinoplasty. This can be achieved by recreating the interdomal ligament with suture and using a transdomal suture for height equalization.[37] If tip maneuvers have caused the LLC to buckle or have an acute bend at the intermediate crura, early bossae will likely be noticeable.

Late bossae are tougher to prevent, especially because they tend to form due to factors beyond the surgeon's control: patients with thin skin and weak LLCs exposed via an external route. The best measure to prevent late bossae in those patients is to perform meticulous undermining in a supraperichondrial plane to prevent postoperative contracture.

Any tip grafting that is misplaced will also lead to the appearance of a bossae, though the deformity is not technically due to an abnormality of the LLC.

## Pinched Tip

The appearance of a pinched tip deformity is self-defining. Although it is necessary to approximate the domes after tip work, excessive narrowing will create the appearance of a pinched tip. This was seen more commonly in the era of vertical dome division but can still occur despite today's principles of tissue conservation with excess dome suturing. The pinched tip can also form due to soft tissue contracture overlying an insufficient tip framework. (**Fig. 11**) For instance, a vertical dome division causes a break in the LLC, leaving the tip to heal on its own postoperatively, and thus at the mercy of contractile scar formation.

To prevent the pinched tip appearance, the cartilaginous framework of the tripod must be reestablished at the end of surgery so that little, if anything, is left to long-term healing. Ideally, reshaping maneuvers can be employed in tip work, and no cartilage resection is necessary. However, should it become necessary to resect portions of the LLC, the tip support mechanisms can be reestablished using columellar struts, interdomal sutures, and tip grafts.[32]

## Excessive Cephalic Rotation

Excessive cephalic rotation is also known as overrotaion. According to the tripod theory of nasal tip support, any surgical maneuver that adds length to the medial crura or shortens the lateral crura will result in over-rotation.[38] (**Fig. 12**) Cephalic overrotaion is not necessarily noticeable to the surgeon at the time of the primary rhinoplasty. Any lateral crura that required shortening may, at the time, appear to provide the appropriate length to the alar limbs of the triangle. However, scarring and contracture in the vector of the resected lateral crura will cause overrotaion of the tip with time. This problem is most commonly seen with an

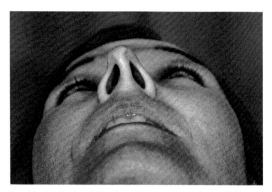

**Fig. 11.** A pinched tip due to over-resection of the tip cartilages and insufficient tip framework.

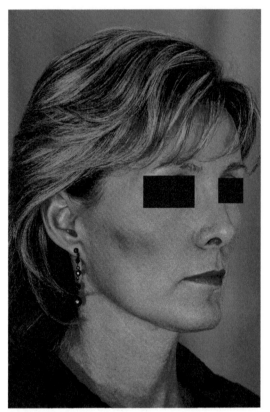

**Fig. 12.** This patient developed excessive cephalic rotation over time after previous rhinoplasty.

excessive cephalic trim of the LLC and vertical dome division, which can be prevented by placing lateral crural strut grafts.[39]

Lowering the septal angle will also cause the effect of over-rotation by cephalically rotating the LLC. Inadvertent cephalic rotation of the medial crura can also be caused by excessive resection of the caudal septum.[12] When performing either of these maneuvers, one must take care when recreating the connection of the medial crura to the residual septum: the new relationship must be guided by the ultimate effect on the tip.

### Tip Ptosis

Tip ptosis (under-rotation) occurs secondarily to loss of tip support. (**Fig. 13**) There are multiple maneuvers that cause the tip of the tripod to drop; they include: a transfixion incision, shortening the medial crura, separation of the LLC from the ULC at the scroll region, and loss of septal or columellar support.

Any of the major tip support mechanisms that require disruption to perform a rhinoplasty must be reestablished at the end of the procedure, such that the tip feels unnaturally firm and

supported.[38,40] Again, depending on which support mechanism requires reconstruction, there are many different grafts, struts, or sutures that are available.[39] The surgeon should not be afraid to use grafts to replace the structural support of cartilage that required resection to obtain the primary rhinoplasty goal. Although it may seem to defeat the purpose of the initial resection, often times the in situ cartilage was malformed and the surgeon has more anatomic control over placement and size of the replacement graft.

### Inadequate Definition

Most of the above complications deal with the structure of the tip. Although structural manipulation is the workhorse of tip rhinoplasty, there are occasional patients whose primary problem is an excess soft tissue envelope. Despite perfect surgical maneuvers intended to narrow the tip, the thick skin carries enough structure itself to leave a persistently bulbous tip as the skin will not contract to follow the intended structural manipulations. This is a complication that is usually predictable in the operating room.

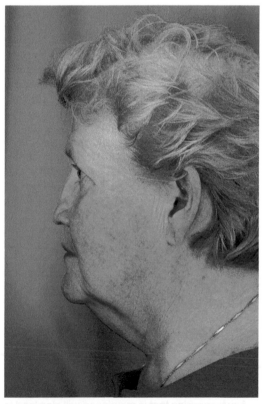

**Fig. 13.** A ptotic tip with loss of projection due to loss of the nasal septum in a patient with Wegener's granulomatosis.

Most of the established teaching in rhinoplasty deals with altering the underlying structure to change the draped appearance of the soft tissue envelope. Excess soft tissue overlying the structure will defeat the purpose of any underlying structural maneuvers, and this is one area where the surgeon must sometimes resect tissue to achieve the desired effect. This can be done meticulously in the lobule and lateral supratip regions. Note, the distal portion of the columellar flap may require excision as it becomes excessive in length after tip retrodisplacement.[41]

## SUMMARY

Rhinoplasty remains one of the most rewarding surgeries performed by facial plastic surgeons. Both surgeons and patients can feel like they have hit a "home run" if everything goes as planned, but there can just as well be mutual disappointment when the outcome differs from expectations. Many of the common complications can be avoided through attention to specific surgical maneuvers during the primary rhinoplasty with deliberate actions, additional grafts, or more conservative resections. Viewing these complications in hindsight can highlight common pitfalls to be considered preemptively at the time of surgery.

## REFERENCES

1. Rothbaum D, Earnest L, Papel ID. Complications in rhinoplasty. In: Becker DG, Park SS, editors. Revision rhinoplasty. New York: Thieme Medical Publishers; 2008. p. 20–31.
2. Quatela VC, Jacono AA. Structural grafting in rhinoplasty. Facial Plast Surg 2002;18:223–32.
3. Mazzola RF, Felisati G. Secondary rhinoplasty: analysis of the deformity and guidelines for management. Facial Plast Surg 1997;13:163–77.
4. Constantinides M, Bustillo A, Shah A. Anatomy and analysis. In: Becker DG, Park SS, editors. Revision rhinoplasty. New York: Thieme Medical Publishers; 2008. p. 3–11.
5. Vuyk HD, Watts SJ, Vindayak B. Revision rhinoplasty: review of deformities, aetiology and treatment strategies. Clin Otolaryngol Allied Sci 2000; 25:476–81.
6. Foda HM. Rhinoplasty for the multiply revised nose. Am J Otolaryngol 2005;26:28–34.
7. Kamer FM, McQuown SA. Revision rhinoplasty. Analysis and treatment. Arch Otolaryngol Head Neck Surg 1988;114:257–66.
8. Foda HM. Management of the droopy tip: a comparison of three alar cartilage-modifying techniques. Plast Reconstr Surg 2003;112:1408–17 [discussion 1418–1].
9. Wright WK. Symposium: the supra-tip in rhinoplasty: a dilemma. II. Influence of surrounding structure and prevention. Laryngoscope 1976;86:50–2.
10. Tardy ME, Brown R. Surgical anatomy of the nose. New York: Raven Press; 1990.
11. Hanasono MM, Kridel RW, Pastorek NJ, et al. Correction of the soft tissue pollybeak using triamcinolone injection. Arch Facial Plast Surg 2002;4: 26–30 [discussion 31].
12. Farrior EH. Revision rhinoplasty for monographs in facial plastic surgery contemporary rhinoplasty. Facial Plast Surg 1997;13:299–308.
13. Gruber R, Chang TN, Kahn D, et al. Broad nasal bone reduction: an algorithm for osteotomies. Plast Reconstr Surg 2007;119:1044–53.
14. Toriumi DM. Rhinoplasty. In: Park SS, editor. Facial plastic surgery: the essential guide. New York: Thieme; 2005. p. 223–53.
15. Arslan E, Aksoy A. Upper lateral cartilage-sparing component dorsal hump reduction in primary rhinoplasty. Laryngoscope 2007;117:990–6.
16. Rohrich RJ, Muzaffar AR, Janis JE. Component dorsal hump reduction: the importance of maintaining dorsal aesthetic lines in rhinoplasty. Plast Reconstr Surg 2004;114:1298–308 [discussion 1309–2].
17. Ballert JA, Park SS. Functional rhinoplasty: treatment of the dysfunctional nasal sidewall. Facial Plast Surg 2006;22:49–54.
18. Neel HB 3rd. Implants of gore-tex. Arch Otolaryngol 1983;109:427–33.
19. Ham J, Miller PJ. Expanded polytetrafluoroethylene implants in rhinoplasty: literature review, operative techniques, and outcome. Facial Plast Surg 2003; 19:331–9.
20. Godin MS, Waldman SR, Johnson CM Jr. Nasal augmentation using gore-tex. A 10-year experience. Arch Facial Plast Surg 1999;1:118–21 [discussion 122].
21. Jin HR, Lee JY, Yeon JY, et al. A multicenter evaluation of the safety of gore-tex as an implant in asian rhinoplasty. Am J Rhinol 2006;20:615–9.
22. Davis PK, Jones SM. The complications of silastic implants. Experience with 137 consecutive cases. Br J Plast Surg 1971;24:405–11.
23. Romo T 3rd, Sclafani AP, Sabini P. Use of porous high-density polyethylene in revision rhinoplasty and in the platyrrhine nose. Aesthetic Plast Surg 1998;22:211–21.
24. Clark JM, Cook TA. Immediate reconstruction of extruded alloplastic nasal implants with irradiated homograft costal cartilage. Laryngoscope 2002; 112:968–74.
25. Raghavan U, Jones NS, Romo T 3rd. Immediate autogenous cartilage grafts in rhinoplasty after alloplastic implant rejection. Arch Facial Plast Surg 2004;6:192–6.

26. Kridel RW, Kraus WM. Grafts and implants in revision rhinoplasty. Facial Plast Surg Clin North Am 1995;3:473–86.

27. Burke AJ, Wang TD, Cook TA. Irradiated homograft rib cartilage in facial reconstruction. Arch Facial Plast Surg 2004;6:334–41.

28. Gryskiewicz JM, Rohrich RJ, Reagan BJ. The use of alloderm for the correction of nasal contour deformities. Plast Reconstr Surg 2001;107:561–70 [discussion 571].

29. Murrell GL. Auricular cartilage grafts and nasal surgery. Laryngoscope 2004;114:2092–102.

30. Kim DW, Shah AR, Toriumi DM. Concentric and eccentric carved costal cartilage: a comparison of warping. Arch Facial Plast Surg 2006;8:42–6.

31. Harshbarger RJ, Sullivan PK. The optimal medial osteotomy: a study of nasal bone thickness and fracture patterns. Plast Reconstr Surg 2001;108: 2114–9 [discussion 2120–1].

32. Constantinides M, Liu ES, Miller PJ, et al. Vertical lobule division in rhinoplasty: maintaining an intact strip. Arch Facial Plast Surg 2001;3: 258–63.

33. Park SS, Becker SS. Repair of nasal airway obstruction in revision rhinoplasty. In: Becker DG, Park SS, editors. Revision rhinoplasty. New York: Thieme; 2008. p. 52–68.

34. Parkes ML, Kanodia R, Machida BK. Revision rhinoplasty. An analysis of aesthetic deformities. Arch Otolaryngol Head Neck Surg 1992;118:695–701.

35. Gillman GS, Simons RL, Lee DJ. Nasal tip bossae in rhinoplasty. etiology, predisposing factors, and management techniques. Arch Facial Plast Surg 1999;1:83–9.

36. Kridel RW, Yoon PJ, Koch RJ. Prevention and correction of nasal tip bossae in rhinoplasty. Arch Facial Plast Surg 2003;5:416–22.

37. Behmand RA, Ghavami A, Guyuron B. Nasal tip sutures part I: the evolution. Plast Reconstr Surg 2003; 112:1125–9 [discussion 1146–9].

38. McCollough EG, Robertson MD, Greco TM. Nasal tip asymmetries. Facial Plast Surg Clin North Am 1995;3:353–66.

39. Toriumi DM. New concepts in nasal tip contouring. Arch Facial Plast Surg 2006;8:156–85.

40. Jang TY, Choi YS, Jung YG, et al. Effect of nasal tip surgery on asian noses using the transdomal suture technique. Aesthetic Plast Surg 2007;31:174–8.

41. Adamson PA, Little JA. Revision tip rhinoplasty. In: Becker DG, Park SS, editors. Revision rhinoplasty. New York: Thieme; 2008. p. 69–84.

# Tissue Engineering for Rhinoplasty

Deborah Watson, MD, FACS

**KEYWORDS**

- Tissue engineering • Human septum
- Cartilage • Tissue culture

Reconstructive surgery of the nose frequently requires re-establishing the form and integrity of the nasal framework, particularly when structural defects of the nose have been created by trauma, previous surgical resection, or congenital anomalies. Autologous, allogenic, and synthetic implants and grafts are the typical materials used in reconstructive rhinoplasty.[1–3] Allogenic materials have a known risk for immune rejection, disease transmission, and resorption, whereas synthetic materials are associated with risks for infection, extrusion, and foreign body reactions.[3] For many rhinoplasty surgeons, autologous tissue (particularly cartilage) tends to be the preferred material, with donor sites from the nasal septum, auricular conchal bowl, and the costal region. Anecdotally, autologous cartilage from the septum is viewed as the ideal cartilage source for repairing cartilaginous and bony nasal defects because of its favorable mechanical properties, ease of harvest, and minimal donor site morbidity. It is firm, nonmalleable, and has superior supportive properties to resist deformity from the contraction of skin and scar during the healing process. These advantages are not apparent with the use of auricular cartilage. The harvesting of costal cartilage entails greater morbidity and is associated with a greater degree of resorption and warping compared with septal cartilage. Unfortunately, the supply of autologous septal cartilage for direct tissue transplantation is limited by the tissue's small size availability and solitary presence in the human body.

A clinical need exists to develop an autologous cartilage tissue supply that can be expanded to the amount required for reconstructive rhinoplasty. Tissue-engineering technology offers the potential to create an abundant quantity of septal cartilage from a small autologous donor specimen. Ideally, the fabricated tissue should resemble native tissue with respect to its biochemical, structural, and metabolic properties. These properties are essential to achieve the appropriate biomechanical function and stability of the replacement tissue in a surgical site.

Tissue engineering is a rapidly developing and expanding interdisciplinary field that applies the principles of engineering and biologic sciences toward the goal of repairing or replacing human tissue. The technology uses cells that are supported in an engineered extracellular matrix and a combination of nutrient factors or molecules. This article describes some of the research methodologies currently used in cartilage tissue engineering that help to optimize the conditions for chondrogenesis, extracellular matrix production, and cartilage construct maturation.

## COMPARISON OF HUMAN CARTILAGE TISSUE TYPES

Septal, auricular, costal, and articular cartilage have all been used for cartilage tissue-engineering studies. Historically, greater emphasis has been placed on studies involving articular cartilage because of the prevalence of research conducted for osteoarthritis. Because there is variability within the biochemical and biomechanical properties of all the cartilage types, it is possible that the methodologies used to engineer a construct with articular chondrocytes may have a different impact on construct fabrication from a different cartilage type—even from the same donor. The tissue-engineering literature contains direct comparisons of the proliferative and chondrogenic potential for

Division of Otolaryngology–Head and Neck Surgery, Facial Plastic and Reconstructive Surgery, UCSD School of Medicine, 3350 La Jolla Village Drive, 112-C, San Diego, CA 92161, USA
E-mail address: debwatson@ucsd.edu

Facial Plast Surg Clin N Am 17 (2009) 157–165
doi:10.1016/j.fsc.2008.09.010
1064-7406/08/$ – see front matter © 2009 Elsevier Inc. All rights reserved.

these tissue sources. An early study[4] showed that there is a greater proliferative effect in monolayer culture of human nasal septal chondrocytes compared with auricular cells. In tissue engineering, the successful proliferation of cells in a monolayer culture is a crucial preliminary step used to increase the total cell count needed for eventual construct formation. Another study[5] made the observation that adult human nasal septal chondrocytes have a superior proliferative and chondrogenic potential compared with human articular chondrocytes, and that the nasal cells proliferated four times faster and produced significantly more extracellular glycosaminoglycan (GAG) and type II collagen than articular cells. Both of these extracellular matrix components are primary indicators of matrix production, and ultimately, construct fabrication. Even with the addition of specific growth factors that are known to enhance cellular proliferation, human nasal septal chondrocytes still proliferate faster than auricular or costal chondrocytes.[6] When redifferentiation—the recovery of the chondrocytic phenotype after monolayer expansion—was assessed in this study by measuring the production of GAG and type II collagen, it was found to be poor in costal chondrocytes. These studies, combined with the relative ease of harvest with low morbidity, imply that human nasal septal chondrocytes are promising for tissue engineering of cartilage constructs to be used in reconstructive surgery of the nose.

## DEDIFFERENTIATION OF CHONDROCYTES

Tissue engineering of cartilage begins with harvesting tissue from a donor, followed by enzymatically digesting the extracellular matrix to isolate the chondrocytes. The chondrocytes are then expanded in a two-dimensional monolayer culture, but during this process the cells assume a fibroblastic characteristic, a process called dedifferentiation.[5,7] When the expanded cells are shifted into a three-dimensional culture arrangement, such as in alginate, agarose, or the polyglycolic/poly-L-lactic acid scaffolds, redifferentiation is induced and production of extracellular matrix can occur.[8–10] At this point, the redifferentiated chondrocyte resumes its typical polygonal, round configuration. It has been observed, however, that the capacity of the cells to redifferentiate and form cartilaginous tissue becomes impaired with increasing levels of expansion or number of passages.[7,10]

## ALGINATE AS A GROWTH SYSTEM

Many cartilage tissue-engineering research groups have routinely suspended their chondrocytes in alginate, as opposed to agarose or the poly scaffolds, as a consistently reliable method to circumvent the problem of cellular dedifferentiation.[11,12] Alginate is a copolymer of L-glucuronic acid and D-mannuronic acid that polymerizes to form a gel in the presence of calcium. Alginate can be easily depolymerized with the addition of a calcium chelator, such as sodium citrate or ethylenediaminetetraacetic acid, thereby releasing chondrocytes with their associated pericellular matrix (also known as cell-associated matrix). Previous studies using articular chondrocytes cultured in alginate beads have shown that these cells secrete a matrix similar to that seen in native human cartilage.[12] Similar findings have been noted for human nasal septal chondrocytes cultured in alginate.[10] These cells form a rim of cell-associated matrix containing high levels of GAG and collagen type II. On depolymerization of alginate beads, this tightly adherent matrix remains associated with the cells.

Masuda and colleagues[13–15] took this a step further and introduced a novel scaffold-free approach of creating articular cartilage constructs, called the alginate-recovered chondrocyte (ARC) method. Chondrocytes are first cultured in alginate under optimal conditions to allow formation of a cell-associated matrix. These cells are then released from the alginate and are seeded onto a semipermeable membrane system for additional culturing time, which allows integration of the cells in a three-dimensional configuration, and formation of a cohesive matrix. Subsequent collaborative work[16] used the ARC method to create neocartilage constructs from human nasal septal chondrocytes. The ARC constructs were found to resemble native cartilage—histologically and grossly—and had structural stability to resist deformation when handled with forceps. The ARC method, therefore, represents a promising technique for creating cartilage constructs without the use of potentially immunogenic scaffold materials.

## SUPPLEMENTING CULTURES WITH GROWTH FACTORS

Numerous articular cartilage studies have used the strategy of adding growth factors to the culture media to promote redifferentiation of the chondrocytic phenotype and production of appropriate extracellular matrix. Insulin-like growth factor–I (IGF-I), fibroblast growth factor (FGF), platelet-derived growth factor (PDGF), the transforming growth factor–β (TGF-β) family, epidermal growth factor (EGF), and members of the bone morphogenetic protein (BMP) superfamily have all been shown to increase proliferation and enhance cartilaginous matrix formation in articular chondrocytes.[17–25]

BMPs are molecules related to the TGF-β superfamily and were originally identified as proteins capable of stimulating endochondral bone formation.[26,27] As potent growth factors, BMPs regulate and modify the differentiation and maturation of various mesenchymal stem cells into osteoblasts, chondroblasts, and adipocytes. More than 47 members of the BMP family have been identified.[28] Among these, BMP-2 and BMP-7 have shown to have stimulatory effects on articular chondrocyte matrix production that exceed those of serum alone.[29–31]

As far as human nasal septal chondrocytes are concerned, TGF-β, FGF-2, IGF-I, PDGF, and BMP-2 have been shown to increase proliferation during two-dimensional monolayer expansion.[4,6,18–22] These early studies did not evaluate the effect of growth factors on human nasal septal cells in three-dimensional culture, but one research group[23] did so using agar. They used serum-free media (SFM) and supplemented it with TGF-β. This growth condition produced more extracellular proteoglycan than with SFM alone. Of note, their cells were not expanded before three-dimensional culture, and therefore they did not succumb to dedifferentiation.

Expansion is necessary to achieve the cell numbers needed to create a large enough cartilage construct for surgical implantation, but expansion typically induces dedifferentiation of the chondrocyte phenotype. Additional steps are required to ensure that redifferentiation occurs. Van Osch and colleagues[24] expanded human nasal septal chondrocytes in monolayer for three or four passages with 10% FBS and then suspended the cells in alginate beads for a three-dimensional culture system to encourage redifferentiation. The alginate-chondrocyte beads were then cultured with SFM or medium supplemented with TGF-β1 and IGF-I. The cells that were exposed to the growth factors produced more GAG and type II collagen. Similarly, Tay and colleagues[6] reported that human septal cells expanded in the presence of TGF-β1, FGF-2, and PDGF-bb for two passages had improved capacity to redifferentiate during three-dimensional culture with TGF-1β and dexamethasone, because dexamethasone has been found to promote chondrocyte differentiation and increase production of IGF-binding proteins.[25] In addition, Hicks and colleagues[32] found a dramatic increase in extracellular matrix production (as measured by a significant increase in GAG production) by human septal chondrocytes, which were expanded in monolayer and then cultured in alginate beads with medium supplemented with FBS, BMP-2, and BMP-7. The combination of BMP-2 and BMP-7 far outperformed either growth factor alone (**Fig. 1**). These studies demonstrate that growth factors can be used to improve redifferentiation by human septal chondrocytes during three-dimensional culture conditions and promote extracellular matrix deposition.

## CARTILAGE TISSUE ENGINEERING WITH HUMAN SERUM

The vast majority of human cartilage tissue-engineering studies published to date have used FBS for serum supplementation. A handful of studies suggest that human serum is superior to FBS for culture of human chondrocytes, however. For articular chondrocytes, human serum has been shown to increase proliferation and production of cartilaginous extracellular matrix relative to FBS.[33–37] Studies by Gruber and colleagues[38] also found an increase in monolayer proliferation of human septal chondrocytes when using autologous human serum. More recently, Chua and colleagues[39] cultured human nasal septal chondrocytes with various concentrations of pooled human serum in addition to FGF, TGF-β2, and IGF-1. They found increased growth rates in monolayer culture with human serum relative to 2% FBS controls. They also described qualitative improvements in mechanical properties and type II collagen in constructs cultured for 8 weeks; however, only limited quantitative data were reported.

Data from another research group[40] supported the finding that human nasal septal chondrocytes expand faster during monolayer culture with pooled human serum compared with FBS controls. In addition, when they transferred their cells to a three-dimensional alginate growth environment, they observed a 3.1-fold higher GAG production with 10% pooled human serum

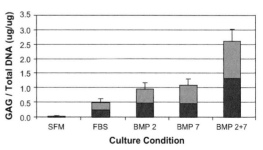

**Fig. 1.** GAG per total DNA in different culture conditions, measuring far-removed matrix (*blue*) and cell-associated matrix (*red*).

compared with 10% FBS. The difference was due to both increased proliferation and increased GAG production per chondrocyte (**Fig. 2**). **Fig. 3** shows Alcian blue staining for one of the samples, demonstrating the increased accumulation of GAG around the cells cultured with higher concentration of human serum. In the 10% and 20% human serum groups, cells and their matrix tended to aggregate in clumps after release from alginate, which is a typical feature of chondrogenic cells. In addition, quantitative assessment for human collagen types I and II was performed with enzyme-linked immunosorbent assay. Total type II collagen production per DNA was more than sixfold higher in each of the human serum groups compared with 10% FBS controls (**Fig. 4**).

Additional studies in this research group supplemented the human sera with the combination of IGF-1 and a BMP growth factor. They observed a greater amount of GAG production, compared with their previous work (**Fig. 5**), and a 12-fold increase in cartilage construct thickness after only 3 weeks of culture (**Fig. 6**). The increase in collagen type II was also more dramatic than with the earlier findings using human sera alone (**Fig. 7**).

These studies suggest that culture in medium supplemented with human serum improves the biochemical properties of tissue-engineered human nasal septal cartilage.

## BIOREACTOR STUDIES

There has been much work on the biomechanical properties of articular cartilage constructs. One research group[41] conducted experiments on articular chondrocytes that were seeded onto polyglycolic acid and poly-L-lactic acid scaffolds. The cells were cultured in a direct perfusion bioreactor at a linear perfusion velocity of 1 μm/s for 4 weeks. They showed a 184% increase in GAG, 155% increase in [3H] proline incorporation, and 118% increase in DNA content (an indicator of cellularity). Other studies[42,43] also observed improvement with their articular constructs when the developing construct was perfused. One of these groups[42] tested a perfusion system at a linear velocity of 10 μm/s (with some flow around the developing cartilage construct), and they were able to form constructs with a composition of 25% GAG and 15% type II collagen, and 60% GAG with no type I collagen (a presence of type I collagen is an extracellular component of fibroblastic cells). The observation of enhanced cellularity and matrix deposition indicate that direct perfusion may improve the properties of neocartilaginous constructs.

In addition, Davisson and colleagues[43] found that constructs subjected to perfusion during culture had significantly higher DNA content (cellularity) than those cultured statically. They also observed that 9 days of continuous perfusion increased GAG synthesis and deposition by approximately 40% when compared with static controls, implying improved chondrogenesis.

Few studies have used perfusion bioreactors for the purposes of nasal septal tissue engineering. Gorti and colleagues[44] observed a more mechanically robust construct with handling when fresh human septal chondrocytes were cultured in a slowly turning lateral vessel bioreactor for 6 weeks compared with constructs cultured in a spinner flask for 14 days; however, no tests were performed to assess their biomechanical properties. Rotter and colleagues[45] also used perfused culture supplemented with FBS at 1 μm/h for 1 and 2 weeks when investigating the degradation of resorbable polymer scaffolds in transplanted cartilage constructs. Indeed, the use of bioreactors in tissue-engineered articular and septal cartilage has been promising, but published reports to date have focused on chondrocytes formed by synthetic scaffolds in FBS and not by alternate three-dimensional growth systems. Currently, studies are being performed to evaluate the efficacy of perfusion for human septal tissue engineering, using a custom-designed bioreactor (**Fig. 8**).

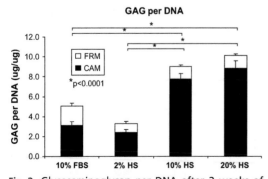

Fig. 2. Glycosaminoglycan per DNA after 2 weeks of culture in alginate beads. The cell-associated matrix (CAM) and far-removed matrix (FRM) components are shown. There was significantly more total GAG production per chondrocyte with 10% human sera (HS) and 20% HS compared with 10% FBS and 2% HS.

## IN VIVO IMPLANTATION OF TISSUE-ENGINEERED CARTILAGE

Cartilage tissue-engineering studies with articular chondrocytes seeded on scaffolds have shown improved histologic features and mechanical

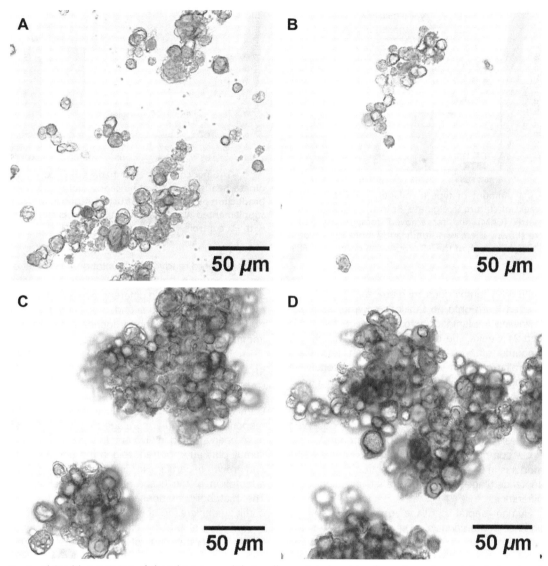

**Fig. 3.** Alcian blue staining of chondrocytes and their cell-associated matrix after release from alginate beads cultured with 10% FBS (*A*), 2% HS (*B*), 10% HS (*C*), or 20% HS (*D*). Strongly positive blue staining indicating GAG accumulation is seen for the 10% and 20% HS groups.

properties after in vivo maturation. Duda and colleagues[46] showed that stiffness and failure load of constructs—fabricated from bovine articular chondrocytes embedded in a fibrinogen/polyglycolic/poly-L-lactic acid polymer scaffold—significantly increased when they were implanted into nude mice for 6 and 12 weeks. Formation of a chondron-like cell matrix with homogenous distribution of chondrocytes was seen on hematoxylin and eosin staining. Presence of GAG and collagen was also observed on histologic analysis following explantation. Similarly, Eyrich and colleagues[47] formed neocartilage from bovine

articular chondrocytes suspended in a fibrin gel by seeding them onto a polycaprolactone-based polyurethane scaffold. Following in vivo maturation in nude mice for 1, 3, and 6 months, homogenous distributions of GAGs and collagen were observed histologically. The constructs precultivated in vitro also contained much higher amounts of extracellular components compared with chondrocytes implanted without precultivation.

Few reports have focused on the in vivo implantation of tissue-engineered human septal cartilage. Rotter and colleagues[45] engineered human septal constructs from human chondrocytes

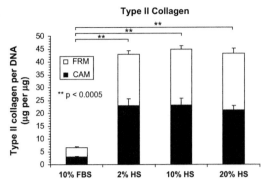

Fig. 4. Amount of type II collagen per DNA after 2 weeks of culture in alginate. Both the cell-associated matrix (CAM) and far-removed components (FRM) are shown. There was significantly more total type II collagen in each of the HS groups compared with FBS.

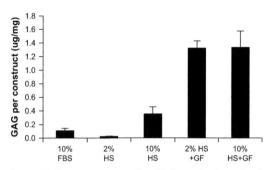

Fig. 5. GAG per construct after 10 days of culture in alginate beads. There is significantly more total GAG production per DNA in constructs cultured in medium supplemented with HS and growth factors compared with HS controls.

cultured in autologous medium and in FBS and seeded them onto an Ethisorb-polymer scaffold. Following implantation into nude mice for 6, 12, and 24 weeks, the constructs showed abundant amounts of type I and II collagen and GAG centrally; collagen was observed peripherally. In another study, Haisch and colleagues[48] implanted polyglycolic/poly-L-lactic acid-polymer scaffolds of human septal cartilage constructs into nude mice for 6 and 12 weeks, and observed synthesis of abundant mucopolysaccharide matrix. A comparison of failure load and compressive modulus in 6- and 12-week constructs and native septal cartilage showed no statistically significant difference.

Human septal cartilage constructs tend to undergo maturation in an in vivo model. As the tissue matures, it achieves a balance between matrix synthesis and degradation such that structural stability and the biomechanical properties typically improve over time. Ideally, when these properties reach levels equivalent to those of native human cartilage, the tissue construct would

be considered ready for implantation. In vivo studies are ongoing that involve varying the in vitro culture conditions with different media and growth factor supplementation, and modifying the time period allotted for chondrogenesis before the immature cartilage construct is implanted.

## SHAPE FIDELITY OF TISSUE-ENGINEERED CARTILAGE CONSTRUCTS

Cartilage is a mechanosensitive tissue, and the responses of articular cartilage to physical forces have been studied in vivo and in vitro. Mechanical stimuli play an important role in the development and growth of cartilage in vivo and in the functional adaptation of the tissue nearing maturation.[49,50] The metabolic responses of chondrocytes and cartilage explants to controlled mechanical stimuli in vitro have also been extensively studied.[51,52] A better understanding of these metabolic responses has encouraged the use of mechanical loading in articular tissue-engineering studies to improve the biochemical and mechanical properties of cartilage constructs.[53] The mechanical behavior and shape fidelity of engineered septal

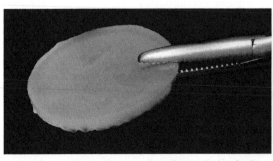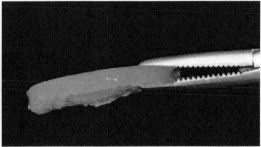

Fig. 6. Representative ARC construct after 3 weeks of culture in 2% HS and growth factor combination. The construct is 12 mm in diameter and 2 mm thick. It exhibits a white, glistening color, similar to native septal cartilage.

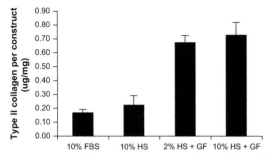

**Fig. 7.** Type II collagen per construct after 10 days of culture in alginate beads. An increase in type II collagen per DNA is seen in constructs cultured in medium supplemented with HS and growth factors relative to HS controls without growth factor supplementation.

cartilage has not been addressed in vitro or in conditions of surgical handling, however. It is necessary to understand what the mechanical environment is of the nasal framework, to fabricate septal cartilage constructs that can withstand the contractile forces of the nasal skin–soft tissue

envelope during the healing process following reconstructive rhinoplasty.

## SUMMARY

Tissue engineering of human septal cartilage can have a profound impact on clinical health care solutions for reconstructive rhinoplasty or, more broadly, craniofacial reconstruction. It would eliminate the health risks and morbidity associated with large cartilage harvesting procedures and the higher rates of infection, rejection, and exposure to transmissible disease when cadaveric or synthetic materials are used. Research in this area is now at a point at which developing human septal cartilage constructs is feasible, but progress is continuing in the efforts to improve chondrogenesis and enhance the maturation of the tissue by manipulating the conditions under which the cartilage constructs grow. Cell metabolism and biosynthesis of the extracellular matrix affect the biomechanical properties of the developing construct, which in turn dictate the structural stability of the tissue. The integrity of the tissue

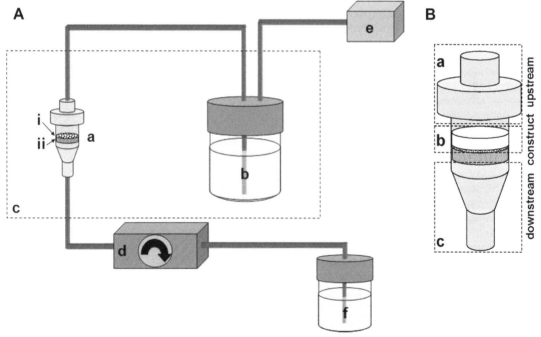

**Fig. 8.** Perfusion bioreactor model. (*A*) The entire system consists of six main components: (a) the bioreactor chamber in which the cells are seeded and the construct is formed on top of (i) the membrane, which is placed on top of (ii) the frit; (b) the media reservoir provides the nutrients for the cells; (c) the waterbath provides the temperature control; (d) the peristaltic pump controls the perfusion rates and drives the flow of the media through the system; (e) the gas source provides pH control for the media; and (f) the collection reservoir, where the spent media is collected after it has passed through the bioreactor chamber. (*B*) The system is divided into three compartments for analysis: (a) upstream, (b) construct, and (c) downstream. The downstream compartment also includes the collection reservoir.

construct and its shape fidelity must be ensured before it can be useful as a surgical implant.

## REFERENCES

1. Tardy ME Jr, Denneny J III, Fritsch MH. The versatile cartilage autograft in reconstruction of the nose and face. Laryngoscope 1985;95:523–33.
2. Komender J, Marczynski W, Tylman D. Preserved tissue allografts in reconstructive surgery. Cell Tissue Bank 2001;2:103–12.
3. Lovice DB, Mingrone MD, Toriumi DM. Grafts and implants in rhinoplasty and nasal reconstruction. Otolaryngol Clin North Am 1999;32:113–41.
4. Quatela VC, Sherris DA, Rosier RN. The human auricular chondrocyte. Responses to growth factors. Arch Otolaryngol Head Neck Surg 1993;119(1):32–7.
5. Kafienah W, Jakob M, Demarteau O, et al. Three-dimensional tissue engineering of hyaline cartilage: comparison of adult nasal and articular chondrocytes. Tissue Eng 2002;8(5):817–26.
6. Tay AG, Farhadi J, Suetterlin R, et al. Cell yield, proliferation, and postexpansion differentiation capacity of human ear, nasal, and rib chondrocytes. Tissue Eng 2004;10(5–6):762–70.
7. Homicz MR, Schumacher BL, Sah RL, et al. Effects of serial expansion of septal chondrocytes on tissue-engineered neocartilage composition. Otolaryngol Head Neck Surg 2002;127(5):398–408.
8. Benya PD, Shaffer JD. Dedifferentiated chondrocytes reexpress the differentiated collagen phenotype when cultured in agarose gels. Cell 1982;30(1):215–24.
9. Homicz MR, Chia SH, Schumacher BL, et al. Human septal chondrocyte redifferentiation in alginate, polyglycolic acid scaffold, and monolayer culture. Laryngoscope 2003;113(1):25–32.
10. Chia SH, Homicz MR, Schumacher BL, et al. Characterization of human nasal septal chondrocytes cultured in alginate. J Am Coll Surg 2005;200(5):691–704.
11. Guo JF, Jourdian GW, MacCallum DK. Culture and growth characteristics of chondrocytes encapsulated in alginate beads. Connect Tissue Res 1989; 19(2–4):277–97.
12. Hauselmann HJ, Aydelotte MB, Schumacher BL, et al. Synthesis and turnover of proteoglycans by human and bovine adult articular chondrocytes cultured in alginate beads. Matrix 1992;12(2):116–29.
13. Masuda K, Hejna M, Thonar EJ-M. Alginate-recovered-chondrocyte method (ARC method): a novel two-step method for the formation of cartilage tissue. Trans Orthop Res Soc 2000;25:620.
14. Masuda K, Miyazaki T, Pfister B, et al. Human tissue engineered cartilage by the alginate-recovered-chondrocyte method after an expansion in monolayer. Trans Orthop Res Soc 2002;27:467.
15. Masuda K, Sah RL, Hejna MJ, et al. A novel two-step method for the formation of tissue engineered cartilage: the alginate-recovered-chondrocyte (ARC) method. J Orthop Res 2003;21(1):139–48.
16. Chia SH, Schumacher BL, Klein TJ, et al. Tissue-engineered human nasal septal cartilage using the alginate-recovered-chondrocyte method. Laryngoscope 2004;114(1):38–45.
17. Masuda K, Pfister BE, Sah RL, et al. Osteogenic protein-1 promotes the formation of tissue-engineered cartilage using the alginate-recovered-chondrocyte method. Osteoarthritis Cartilage 2006;14(4):384–91.
18. Vetter U, Zapf J, Henrichs I, et al. Human nasal septal cartilage: analysis of intracellular enzyme activities, glycogen content, cell density and clonal proliferation of septal chondrocytes of healthy adults and acromegalic patients. Connect Tissue Res 1989;18(4):243–54.
19. Bujia J, Sittinger M, Wilmes E, et al. Effect of growth factors on cell proliferation by human nasal septal chondrocytes cultured in monolayer. Acta Otolaryngol 1994;114(5):539–43.
20. Dunham BP, Koch RJ. Basic fibroblast growth factor and insulinlike growth factor I support the growth of human septal chondrocytes in a serum-free environment. Arch Otolaryngol Head Neck Surg 1998; 124(12):1325–30.
21. Lavezzi A, Mantovani M, della Berta LG, et al. Cell kinetics of human nasal septal chondrocytes in vitro: importance for cartilage grafting in otolaryngology. J Otolaryngol 2002;31(6):366–70.
22. Richmon JD, Sage AB, Shelton E, et al. Effect of growth factors on cell proliferation, matrix deposition, and morphology of human nasal septal chondrocytes cultured in monolayer. Laryngoscope 2005;115(9):1553–60.
23. Bujia J, Pitzke P, Kastenbauer E, et al. Effect of growth factors on matrix synthesis by human nasal chondrocytes cultured in monolayer and in agar. Eur Arch Otorhinolaryngol 1996;253(6):336–40.
24. van Osch GJ, Marijnissen WJ, van der Veen SW, et al. The potency of culture-expanded nasal septum chondrocytes for tissue engineering of cartilage. Am J Rhinol 2001;15(3):187–92.
25. Nadra R, Menuelle P, Chevallier S, et al. Regulation by glucocorticoids of cell differentiation and insulin-like growth factor binding protein production in cultured fetal rat nasal chondrocytes. J Cell Biochem 2003;88(5):911–22.
26. Sampath TK, Reddi AH. Dissociative extraction and reconstitution of extracellular matrix components involved in local bone differentiation. Proc Natl Acad Sci U S A 1981;78:7599–603.
27. Urist MR, Mikulski A, Lietze A. Solubilized and insolubilized bone morphogenetic protein. Proc Natl Acad Sci U S A 1979;76:1828–32.
28. Chubinskaya S, Kuettner KE. Regulation of osteogenic proteins by chondrocytes. Int J Biochem Cell Biol 2003;35:1323–40.

29. Flechtenmacher J, Huch K, Thonar EJ, et al. Recombinant human osteogenic protein 1 is a potent stimulator of the synthesis of cartilage proteoglycans and collagens by human articular chondrocytes. Arthritis Rheum 1996;39:1896–904.

30. Nishida Y, Knudson CB, Eger W, et al. Osteogenic protein-1 stimulates cell-associated matrix assembly by normal human articular chondrocytes: upregulation of hyaluronan synthase. Arthritis Rheum 2000; 43:206–14.

31. Sailor LZ, Hewick RM, Morris EA. Recombinant human bone morphogenetic protein-2 maintains the articular chondrocyte phenotype in long-term culture. J Orthop Res 1996;14:937–45.

32. Hicks DL, Sage AB, Shelton E, et al. Effect of bone morphogenetic proteins 2 and 7 on septal chondrocytes in alginate. Otolaryngol Head Neck Surg 2007; 136(3):373–9.

33. Choi YC, Morris GM, Lee FS, et al. The effect of serum on monolayer cell culture of mammalian articular chondrocytes. Connect Tissue Res 1980;7:105–12.

34. Ostensen M, Veiby OP, Raiss R. Responses of normal and rheumatic human articular chondrocytes cultured under various experimental conditions in agarose. Scand J Rheumatol 1991;20:172–82.

35. Anderer U, Libera J. In vitro engineering of human autogenous cartilage. J Bone Miner Res 2002;17: 1420–9.

36. Badrul AH, Aminuddin BS, Sharaf I, et al. The effects of autologous human serum on the growth of tissue engineered human articular cartilage. Med J Malaysia 2004;59(Suppl B):11–2.

37. Tallheden T, van der Lee J, Brantsing C, et al. Human serum for culture of articular chondrocytes. Cell Transplant 2005;14:469–79.

38. Gruber R, Sittinger M, Bujia J. [In vitro cultivation of human chondrocytes using autologous human serum supplemented culture medium: minimizing possible risk of infection with pathogens of prion diseases]. Laryngorhinootologie 1996;75(2):105–8.

39. Chua KH, Aminuddin BS, Fuzina NH, et al. Human serum provided additional values in growth factors supplemented medium for human chondrocytes monolayer expansion and engineered cartilage construction. Med J Malaysia 2004;59(Suppl B):194–5.

40. Alexander T, Sage BS, Schumacher B, et al. Human serum for tissue engineering of human nasal septal cartilage. Otolaryngol Head Neck Surg 2006;135: 397–403.

41. Pazzano D, Mercier KA, Moran JM, et al. Comparison of chondrogenesis in static and perfused bioreactor culture. Biotechnol Prog 2000;16(5):893–6.

42. Wu F, Dunkelman N, Peterson A, et al. Bioreactor development for tissue-engineered cartilage. Ann N Y Acad Sci 1999;18(875):405–11.

43. Davisson TH, Sah RL, Ratcliffe AR. Perfusion increases cell content and matrix synthesis in chondrocyte three-dimensional cultures. Tissue Eng 2000;8:807–16.

44. Gorti GK, Lo J, Falsafi S, et al. Cartilage tissue engineering using cryogenic chondrocytes. Arch Otolaryngol Head Neck Surg 2003;129:889–93.

45. Rotter N, Aigner J, Naumann A. Behavior of tissue-engineered human cartilage after transplantation into nude mice. J Mater Sci Mater Med 1999;10: 689–93.

46. Duda GN, Haisch A, endres M, et al. Mechanical quality of tissue engineered cartilage: results after 6 and 12 weeks in vivo. J Biomed Mater Res 2000; 53(96):673–7.

47. Eyrich D, Wiese H, Maier G, et al. In vitro and in vivo cartilage engineering using a combination of chondrocyte-seeded long term stable fibrin gels and polycaprolactone-based polyurethane scaffolds. Tissue Eng 2007;13(9):2207–18.

48. Haisch A, Duda GN, Schroeder D, et al. The morphology and biomechanical characteristics of subcutaneously implanted tissue engineered human septal cartilage. Eur Arch Otorhinolaryngol 2005; 262:993–7.

49. Kiviranta I, Tammi M, Jurvelin J, et al. Moderate running exercise augments glycosaminoglycans and thickness of articular cartilage in the knee joint of young beagle dogs. J Orthop Res 1988;6:188–95.

50. Plochocki JH, Riscigno CJ, Garcia M. Functional adaptation of the femoral head to voluntary exercise. Anat Rec A Discov Mol Cell Evol Biol 2006;288:776–81.

51. Guilak F, Sah RL, Setton LA. Physical regulation of cartilage metabolism. In: Mow VC, Hayes WC, editors. Basic orthopaedic biomechanics. New York: Raven Press; 1997. p. 179–207.

52. Grodzinsky AJ, Levenston ME, Jin M, et al. Cartilage tissue remodeling in response to mechanical forces. Annu Rev Biomed Eng 2000;2:691–713.

53. Guilak F, Butler DL, Goldstein SA. Functional tissue engineering: the role of biomechanics in articular cartilage repair. Clin Orthop Relat Res 2001;391(Suppl): 295–305.

# Index

*Note:* Page numbers of article titles are in **boldface** type.

# *Moving?*

## *Make sure your subscription moves with you!*

To notify us of your new address, find your **Clinics Account Number** (located on your mailing label above your name), and contact customer service at:

E-mail: elspcs@elsevier.com

800-654-2452 (subscribers in the U.S. & Canada)
314-453-7041 (subscribers outside of the U.S. & Canada)

Fax number: 314-523-5170

**Elsevier Periodicals Customer Service**
11830 Westline Industrial Drive
St. Louis, MO 63146

*To ensure uninterrupted delivery of your subscription, please notify us at least 4 weeks in advance of move.

Printed and bound by CPI Group (UK) Ltd, Croydon, CR0 4YY

03/10/2024

01040363-0019